FLUIDS AND ELECTROLYTES—
THE GUIDE FOR EVERYDAY PRACTICE
THE LITTLE YELLOW BOOK

FREDERICK C. WHITTIER, M.D.
GREGORY W. RUTECKI, M.D.

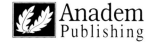

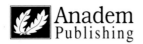

3620 North High Street
Columbus, OH 43214
Tel: 1 (800) 633-0055

Fluids and Electrolytes; The Guide for Everyday Practice:
The Little Yellow Book
Frederick C. Whittier, M.D.
Gregory W. Rutecki, M.D.

The chapters in this book were previously published in *Consultant* and the *Journal of Critical Illness* and are reprinted with permission of the Cliggott Publishing Co., 55 Holly Hill Lane, Box 4010, Greenwich, CT 06831-0010. The authors have updated the content for this book.

PRINTED IN THE UNITED STATES OF AMERICA

ISBN 1-890018-33-3

PREFACE

Both authors sympathize with clinicians who struggle through the acid-base and fluid-electrolyte problems complicating everyday practice. Although we ourselves have served as consultants, believe it or not, we have had our own difficulties learning the essential tools of problem-solving in renal physiology. Many of our former mentors approached problem-solving in this arena by gestalt and were unable to share their expertise with students and residents. We feel strongly that this important area of clinical medicine can be simplified, and that apparently complex problems are solvable with a valid, reproducible, and systematic approach. This book is our humble attempt to teach clinical problem-solving skills in the exciting area of acid-base and fluid-electrolyte physiology. We hope you enjoy our efforts.

Frederick C. Whittier, M.D.

Gregory W. Rutecki, M.D.

Using This Book

Publisher's Notes

TABLE OF CONTENTS

1. Acid-Base Interpretation
Part I: Applying Five Rules in Everyday Cases

Must primary care physicians be "fluent" in acid-base physiology? Yes, for two major reasons:

First, many common disease states can become evident through acid-base disorders. Patients with early septicemia, for example, may initially have only a respiratory alkalemia.

Second, some rarer diseases become suspect when you observe abnormalities in acid-base status. For example, a rheumatic disease such as Sjögren's syndrome may be diagnosed by means of a nonanion gap acidemia. Multiple myeloma may cause a decreased or absent anion gap. Primary aldosterone excess, a rare cause of hypertension, may make itself known through a combined hypokalemia and metabolic alkalemia. The development of an anion gap in a patient who has a mixed acid-base disorder may lead to the diagnosis of lactic acidosis, which portends a more severe illness.

Fortunately, the reputed complexity of interpreting acid-base disorders can be greatly simplified. Here we present five rules for interpreting clinical acid-base physiology and sample cases in which these rules are applied. This methodical five-point scheme will also help you solve more complex cases of acid-base disorders, such as mixed and triple acid-base disturbances, as we will demonstrate in the next chapter.

The Five Rules

Homeostasis of the human body demands that hydrogen ions in body fluids be precisely regulated. The regulation, or **acid-base balance**, relies on lung and kidney adjustments — for carbon dioxide and a bicarbonate balance, respectively — that will maintain the chemical environment optimal for cellular function.

Fact-finding begins with obtaining an arterial blood gas analysis and a serum electrolyte measurement. We will use these numbers in the formulas presented in the Five Rules.

The arterial blood gas sample provides the pH, the partial pressures of carbon dioxide (PCO_2) and oxygen (PO_2), and the bicarbonate level. These help identify both the primary acid-base situation and the body's attempt to compensate.

Electrolytes in a serum sample drawn near the time of the blood-gas determination give the values to calculate the anion gap.

1. Use the Blood Gas to Determine Whether Acidemia or Alkalemia is Present

A normal serum pH is 7.40 to 7.44. Any pH less than 7.40 represents acidemia; any pH greater than 7.44 indicates alkalemia. Thus, alkalemia and acidemia cannot exist simultaneously. It is a mistake to use the terms "acidemia" and "acidosis" or "alkalemia" and "alkalosis" interchangeably. Doing so could obscure the fact that a patient may have a significant underlying acidosis without acidemia, or alkalosis without alkalemia.

For example, a patient with pH 7.46 would be considered to have alkalemia. If this patient simultaneously has an anion gap elevation, there would be an anion gap acidosis but not acidemia. Another patient might initially have a normal pH or even an acidemia but a markedly decreased PCO_2 consistent with a respiratory alkalosis. Thus, a patient can have an alkalosis without alkalemia.

Remember, too, that primary metabolic processes can have numerous causes. Metabolic alkalemia may result from vomiting or from mineralocorticoid excess with hydrogen ion loss from the kidneys. Metabolic acidemia may result from diarrhea, renal tubular disease, or excess acid ingestion or production.

Therefore, in any clinical situation, it is possible to have two or more primary metabolic processes operational. The lung, however, is the *only* organ responsible for the respiratory acid-base status. Because a patient cannot breathe too much and too little simultaneously, only one respiratory process can be present at any given time.

2. When Acidemia or Alkalemia is Found, Determine Whether this Primary Process is Respiratory or Metabolic

Alkalemia (pH greater than 7.44) has an underlying **respiratory** cause if the PCO_2 is substantially less than 40 mm Hg. It has a **metabolic** cause if the bicarbonate content is greater than 26 mEq/L. When the PCO_2 is less than 40 mmHg at the same time that bicarbonate is greater than 26 mEq/L, primary respiratory alkalemia and metabolic alkalemia may coexist (normal bicarbonate range varies slightly among labs).

A new range for a normal anion gap

Since calculation of the serum anion gap is the critical branch point in determining the presence and cause of metabolic acidosis, an accurate normal reference range is essential. The concept of the anion gap arose from the principle of electroneutrality in 1939, when Gamble observed that the positive and negative charges in serum must be balanced. The range for normal was verified initially in the 1970s as 12 ± 4 (8 to 16 mEq/L).

In reality, the so-called gap is caused by a variety of unmeasured anions and cations (albumin, organic anions, phosphate, sulfate, potassium, calcium, and magnesium). Since there are more measured cations, the gap is due to unmeasured anions.

The verification of a normal range for anion gap occurred in an era when flame photometry was the gold standard for serum electrolyte determinations. Within the last few years, a transition has occurred away from flame photometry to the use of ion-specific electrodes. Compared with flame photometry, the electrodes have a chloride bias, in that chloride measurements are consistently 2 to 6 mEq/L higher. This chloride overestimation has lowered the range for normal anion gap reference values. Recent investigators have offered a new range for the anion gap at 6.6 ± 4 (2.6 to 10.6 mEq/L).

The key to interpreting anion gaps correctly in the evaluation of acid-base disorders is to know the reference values for each specific laboratory. Clinicians must be aware that the contemporary reference value may not be the traditional 12 mEq/L.

It is also imperative to realize that a 1g drop in albumin leads to a 2.5 drop in normal anion gap. Since albumin is a substantial proportion of the unmeasured anions, this is not surprising. Therefore, a seemingly normal gap of 10 corrected with a 2g decrease in albumin actually represents an anion gap of 15 (2g decrease in albumin = 5 drop in anion gap) and may indicate underlying metabolic acidosis.

Acidemia (pH less than 7.40) has an underlying **respiratory** cause if the PCO_2 is greater than 40 mm Hg. It has an underlying **metabolic** cause if the bicarbonate content is less than 25 mEq/L. However, if the PCO_2 is greater than 40 mm Hg and the bicarbonate less than 25 mEq/L, a primary respiratory acidemia and metabolic acidemia may coexist.

3. Always Calculate the Anion Gap

The anion gap is the difference between the concentrations of serum cations and anions, determined by measuring the concentrations of sodium cations and bicarbonate and chloride anions (see "A New Range for a Normal Anion Gap"). We calculate it by subtracting the sum of the serum bicarbonate and chloride concentrations from that of serum sodium. The normal anion gap is 10 mEq/L, with a range between 3 mEq/L and 12 mEq/L.

- An anion gap greater than 12 mEq/L can identify a metabolic acidosis. If the anion gap exceeds 20 mEq/L, metabolic acidosis always exists, by definition.

- A gap less than 3 mEq/L, with or without an acid-base disturbance, raises suspicion of conditions as diverse as multiple myeloma, nephrotic syndrome, bromism, lithium intoxication, and hypoalbuminemia.

4. Always Check for the Degree of Compensation

"Compensation" refers to the fact that the body attenuates any physiologic change by making adjustments that move in a direction opposite the change. For every addition of acid it receives, the body attempts to bring the pH back toward normal by an addition of base. As metabolic alkalemia develops, for example, the body compensates by increasing the amount of respiratory acid in the body (hypoventilation). However, this attempted compensation never fully corrects the primary disturbance.

If the primary process is metabolic, the body's compensation will be respiratory. If the primary process is respiratory, the body's compensation will be metabolic.

Compensation in metabolic acidemia. In metabolic acidemia, the compensatory respiratory change — hyperventilation — results in a lower PCO_2. There are two chief ways to check for compensation:

- In an emergency, the fastest way to "eyeball" compensation for metabolic acidemia is this: the decrease in PCO_2 should equal the last two digits of the pH. In a pure metabolic acidemia, if the pH is 7.20, the PCO_2 should be approximately 20 mm Hg, and this would be a normally compensated metabolic acidemia.

- A more accurate check for compensation is this: the decrease in PCO_2 should equal 1.3 times the decrease in bicarbonate. Thus, in metabolic acidemia, if the bicarbonate decreases to 15 from 25 mEq/L (decrease of 10), the PCO_2 should decrease to 27 mm Hg from 40 mm Hg: ie, $40 - (1.3 \times 10) = 27$. This would indicate appropriate respiratory compensation for metabolic acidemia. In this example, if the PCO_2 were above 30 mm Hg, an additional primary respiratory acidosis would be present; if the PCO_2 were below 24 mm Hg, a primary respiratory alkalosis would be present simultaneously.

We prefer the second method for checking compensation, for reasons that will be clearer after you have read the following discussion.

Compensation in metabolic alkalemia. The body compensates for metabolic increases in bicarbonate (base, alkali) by acid retention by the lung (hypoventilation, with an increase in PCO_2). An obvious drawback to this as a form of compensation is the potential for hypoxemia. The compensatory variable increase in PCO_2 can be estimated as follows: the increase in PCO_2 should equal 0.6 times the increase in bicarbonate level.

To illustrate: If bicarbonate increases to 35 mEq/L from a normal of 25 mEq/L, the appropriate compensation for the PCO_2 is 46 mm Hg: ie, $40 + (0.6 \times 10) = 46$. In this instance, if the PCO_2 is significantly greater than 46 mm Hg, an additional primary respiratory acidosis is present; if the PCO_2 is significantly less than 46, a primary respiratory alkalosis is present.

Compensation for respiratory acidemia and alkalemia. Respiratory acidemia is due to hypoventilation with retention of carbon dioxide. Respiratory alkalemia is due to hyperventilation with a decrease in carbon dioxide. The degree of compensation varies according to whether the situation is acute (2-3 days or less) or chronic.

In the acute stage, respiratory acidemia or alkalemia is countered by an increase or decrease in bicarbonate, which represents the work of the bicarbonate buffer system. If the respiratory disorder is not corrected within 2-3 days, the kidney begins to compensate further for the respiratory situation by the addition or removal of acid or base. In chronic respiratory acidemia, the kidney manufactures and retains bicarbonate. In respiratory alkalemia, the kidney decreases the production of bicarbonate and increases the urinary excretion of bicarbonate.

In the respiratory acidemias and alkalemias, if the calculation of the degree of metabolic compensation is not close to the actual value for the bicarbonate ($\pm$ 2 mEq/L), a primary additional metabolic acidosis or alkalosis is present. (Table 1.1)

5. There Should be a 1:1 Relationship of Acid-base

This concept relies on the basic premise that there can never be an excess of positive or negative charges in the blood. If the cations remain constant at any time and an acid anion is added to the blood, there should be an appropriate and balanced decline in bicarbonate. Calculation of this ratio can help you identify an underlying metabolic alkalosis not detected by application of the previous rules.

In an **increased** anion gap metabolic acidemia, for every 1-point increase in the anion gap, there should be a 1mEq/L decline in the bicarbonate level. A decline in bicarbonate level of less than the increase in the anion gap suggests an underlying metabolic alkalosis. In essence, the bicarbonate level is higher than expected for the increased anion gap because "hidden" metabolic alkalosis means serum bicarbonate started at a higher level (eg, 30 mEq/L rather than 25 mEq/L).

In a **normal** anion gap acidosis, for every 1mEq/L increase in chloride, there should be a 1mEq/L decrease in bicarbonate. Again, if the decline in bicarbonate is less than the increase in chloride, an additional primary metabolic alkalosis is present. In our experience, the 1:1 relationship holds only for the detection of an underlying metabolic alkalosis. If a primary metabolic alkalosis or alkalemia has been determined by use of the first four rules, the 1:1 calculation is unnecessary.

These Five Rules of clinical acid-base physiology should become clear in the context of three representative cases of simple acid-base disorders. Refer to Table 1-1 for related definitions, values, and formulas.

Case 1-1. Metabolic Acidosis Resulting from Laxative Abuse

A 60-year-old woman complains of weakness and fatigue for 1 week. She reluctantly admits to using laxatives because of constipation and has had considerable diarrhea in the last month. There is no significant past medical history, and the physical examination findings are normal. Initial laboratory data include:

> Sodium, 133 mEq/L
> Potassium, 2.8 mEq/L
> Chloride, 118 mEq/L
> pH, 7.26
> PCO_2, 13 mm Hg
> Bicarbonate, 5 mEq/L

Use the five clinical rules to characterize the acid-base disorder:

1. **Acidemia** is present (pH less than 7.40).

2. The primary process is **metabolic** (bicarbonate is decreased to 5 mEq/L, and PCO_2 is not increased).

3. **Anion gap** is normal: $133 - (118 + 5) = 10$.

4. **Compensation.** In primary metabolic acidemia, the formula that checks for compensation is: change in PCO_2 = 1.3 x change in bicarbonate. Here the calculation is: change in PCO_2 = 1.3 × $(25 - 5)$. Therefore, change in PCO_2 = 26; the predicted PCO_2

is 14 (40 − 26 = 14).
The actual PCO_2 is 13 mm Hg, and the predicted PCO_2 is 14 mm Hg. Therefore, the compensation is normal.

5. **1:1 Relationship.** The bicarbonate decrease is 20, ie, 25 − 5 = 20; and the chloride increase is 18, ie, 118 − 100 = 18. The change of 20 vs 18 is within the limits of variability. Therefore, there is no underlying metabolic alkalosis.

We conclude from the rules that this patient has a simple acid-base disturbance, a metabolic acidemia with a normal anion gap. This situation was likely caused by the diarrhea (bicarbonate loss) from the laxative abuse.

Case 1-2. Acute Respiratory Alkalosis with Sepsis

A 74-year-old nursing home resident is admitted to the hospital with hypotension (96/70 mm Hg) and and a temperature of 38.7°C (101.7°F). His urine culture was positive for *Escherichia coli* and two blood cultures were positive for the same organism. The laboratory values are:

Sodium, 137 mEq/L
Potassium, 3.2 mEq/L
Chloride, 105 mEq/L
pH, 7.49
PCO_2, 25mm Hg
Bicarbonate, 22 mEq/L

Use the five clinical rules to characterize the acid-base disorder:

1. **Alkalemia** is present (pH greater than 7.44).

2. The primary process is **respiratory** (PCO_2 less than 40 mm Hg, and bicarbonate is not increased).

3. **Anion gap** is normal: 137 − (105 + 22) = 10.

4. **Compensation.** The decrease in PCO_2 is 40 − 25, or 15. The formula for a decrease in bicarbonate is 2 for every 10 decrease in the PCO_2 (see Table 1-1). In this instance, the calculated decrease is 3 — identical to the actual decrease (ie, 25 − 22 = 3). Therefore, the compensation is normal.

5. **1:1 Relationship.** Since the anion gap is normal, the bicarbonate decrease of 3 (ie, 25 − 22 = 3) is close enough to the chloride increase of 5 (ie, 105 − 100 = 5). Therefore, no underlying metabolic alkalosis exists.

Table 1-1. Key definitions and formulas for interpreting clinical acid-base physiology

Normal values for acid-base determinations
Blood

        pH: 7.40 − 7.44

        PCO_2: 40 mm Hg

        Cations: Sodium: 140 meq/L

        Potassium: 4 meq/l

        Anions: Bicarbonate: 25 meq/L (may vary with different labs)

        Chloride: 100 meq/L

        Anion gap: 3 - 12 with ion-selective electrodes

Rule 1. Determine pH status (alkalemia or acidemia)

Rule 2. Determine whether the primary process is respiratory or metabolic (or both)

Alkalemia

    Respiratory alkalosis: If PCO_2 substantially less than 40 mm Hg

    Metabolic alkalosis: if bicarbonate greater than 25 meq/L

Acidemia

    Respiratory acidemia: if PCO_2 greater than 40 meq/L

    Metabolic acidosis: if bicarbonate less than 25 meq/L

Rule 3. Calculate the serum anion gap

Anion gap = Sodium - (Bicarbonate + Chloride)

- Anion gap that is increased (greater than 12 meq/L) can indicate metabolic acidosis
- Anion gap increased beyond 20 meq/L always indicates a metabolic acidosis

Rule 4. Check the degree of compensation

Metabolic acidosis

    Decrease in PCO_2 = 1.3 ´ decrease in bicarbonate

Metabolic alkalosis

    Increase in PCO_2 = 0.6 ´ increase in bicarbonate

Respiratory acidosis

    Acute: for every PCO_2 increase of 10 m Hg, bicarbonate increases by 1 meq/L

    Chronic: for every PCO_2 increase of 10 mm Hg, bicarbonate increases by 4 meq/L

Respiratory alkalosis

    Acute: for every PCO_2 decrease of 10 mm Hg, bicarbonate decreases by 2 meq/L

    Chronic: for every PCO_2 decrease of 10 mm Hg, bicarbonate decreases by 4 meq/L

Rule 5. Determine whether there is a 1:1 relationship between anions in blood

    Increased anion gap metabolic acidosis: every 1 point increase in anion gap should be accompanied by a 1 meq/L decrease in bicarbonate

    Normal anion gap metabolic acidosis: every 1 meq/L increase in chloride should be accompanied by a 1 meq/L decrease in bicarbonate

This patient has a simple acute respiratory alkalemia. This would be expected and is most commonly seen with sepsis (*E. coli* positive blood culture). Because blood cultures take time to grow, an acute respiratory alkalemia on admission may be the only clue to septicemia!

CASE 1-3. Respiratory Acidosis from Chronic Lung Disease

A 52-year-old male smoker known to have chronic obstructive pulmonary disease is in stable condition when he visits the clinic for a 6 month checkup. Routine laboratory results include these:

> Sodium, 136 mEq/L
> Potassium, 3.8 mEq/L
> Chloride, 92 mEq/L
> pH, 7.34
> PCO_2, 65 mm Hg
> Bicarbonate, 34 mEq/L

Use the five clinical rules to characterize the acid-base disorder:

1. **Acidemia** is present (pH less than 7.40).

2. Primary process is **respiratory** (PCO_2 greater than 40, bicarbonate is not decreased).

3. **Anion gap** is normal: $136 - (92 + 34) = 10$.

4. **Compensation.** In this chronic respiratory acidemia, the PCO_2 is increased 25 (ie, $65 - 40 = 25$). The formula for compensation is that for each increase of 10 mm Hg in the PCO_2, there is an increase of 4 in bicarbonate (see Table 1-1). The calculated compensation is for the bicarbonate to be 35 ($2.5 \times 4 = 10$). Since the measured bicarbonate is 34 mEq/L, the compensation is close enough to the calculated figure, and an underlying primary metabolic process is not present. The compensation is normal.

5. **1:1 Relationship.** Strictly speaking, it is not necessary to calculate this relationship because Rule 4, determining compensation, did not detect an underlying metabolic alkalosis. In this situation, chloride is down 8 mEq/L, and bicarbonate is up 9mEq/L, an appropriate response.

We conclude that this patient has a simple chronic respiratory acidemia caused by the chronic lung disease.

"Take-Home" Message

We recommend that physicians hone their skills using these concepts by preparing a 3 × 5 card that contains the Five Rules and the formulas for the anion gap, compensation, and 1:1 relationship. With the routine of calculating acid base systematically, the rules become an integral component of clinical skills, and the card becomes unnecessary.

Suggested Readings

1.   Duncan A, Morris AJ, Cameron A, et al. Laxative-induced diarrhea — a neglected diagnosis. *J R Soc Med.* 1992;85:203-205.

2.   Gamble JL. *Chemical Anatomy, Physiology, and Pathology of Extracellular Fluids: A Lecture Syllabus.* 6th ed. Cambridge, Mass: Harvard University Press; 1960:131.

3.   Sadjadi SA. A new range for the anion gap. *Ann Intern Med.* 1995;123:807.

4.   Winter SD, Pearson JR, Gabow PA, et al. The fall of the serum anion gap. *Arch Intern Med.* 1990;150: 311-313.

5.   Iberti TJ, Leibowitz AB, Papadakos Pj, et al. Low sensitivity of the anion gap as a screen to detect hyperlactatemia in critically ill patients. *Crit Care Med.* 1990;18:275-278.

6.   Paulson WD. How to interpret the anion gap. *J Crit Illness.* 1997;12:96-99.

7.   Paulson WD. Effect of acute pH change on serum anion gap. *J Am Soc Nephrol.* 1996;7:357-363.

8.   Figge J, Mydosh T, Fencl V. Serum proteins and acid-base equilibria: a follow-up. *J Lab Clin Med.* 1992;120:713-719.

2. Acid-Base Interpretation
Part II: Applying Five Rules to Simplify Complex Cases

In the previous chapter, five rules were introduced for interpreting clinical acid-base physiology. Routine application of these rules will help you solve even complex acid-base disturbances.

Here we present four cases of patients with mixed and triple acid-base disturbances. Our goal is to show how application of the five rules can help you make sense of the data and map out a sound management strategy.

CASE 2-1. Patient with Persistent Vomiting and Severe Liver Disease

A 50-year-old house painter with alcoholic cirrhosis is admitted to the hospital after several days of abdominal pain and vomiting. Physical examination reveals confusion, asterixis, and ascites. Supine blood pressure is 106/78 mm Hg; upright blood pressure is 104/60 mm Hg. Initial laboratory data include the following values:

> Sodium, 126 mEq/L
> Potassium, 2.8 mEq/L
> Chloride, 80 mEq/L
> pH, 7.60
> PCO_2, 34 mm Hg
> Bicarbonate, 36 mEq/L

Use the five clinical rules to characterize the acid-base disorder (Table 1-1):

1. **Alkalemia is present** (pH is greater than 7.44).

2. The primary process is both **metabolic** (bicarbonate is increased to 36 mEq) and *respiratory* (the PCO_2 is decreased to 34 mm Hg).

3. The **anion gap** is normal:
$$126 - (80 + 36) = 10.$$

4. **Compensation.** Recall that in primary metabolic alkalemia,

the formula that checks for compensation is: change in PCO_2 = 0.6 × increase in bicarbonate. Since the change in bicarbonate is 11 (bicarbonate increased to 36 mEq/L from 25 mEq/L), the change in PCO_2 should be an increase of 6.6 (11 × 0.6) and should result in a PCO_2 of about 47 (40 + 6.6 = 47). The actual PCO_2 of 34 mm Hg, which is much less than predicted, defines a second primary process of respiratory alkalosis.

5. **1:1 Relationship.** In this case, you need not calculate this relationship since a metabolic alkalemia has already been established.

This patient has a mixed acid-base disturbance: a metabolic alkalemia and a respiratory alkalosis. The metabolic alkalemia is most likely due to his persistent vomiting with loss of acid from the stomach. Many patients with severe liver disease will have a primary respiratory alkalosis of unknown etiology as seen in this patient. Indeed, severe liver disease is second only to septicemia on the list of causes of respiratory alkalosis.

Differential diagnosis of metabolic alkalosis. The recommended approach relies on information from a spot urinary chloride measurement:

Patients with metabolic alkalosis and a low urinary chloride level (less than 10 mEq/L) have volume contraction and therefore respond to normal saline with correction of metabolic alkalosis; their condition is designated **saline responsive.**

Patients with metabolic alkalosis and high urinary chloride level (usually greater than 20 mEq/L) are not volume contracted; their condition is, therefore, termed **saline resistant.** Most patients in this category have an excess of either mineralocorticoid or glucocorticoid hormone.

The urinary chloride test is more sensitive and specific than that for urinary sodium, and the results of this test should be considered before treatment decisions are made in cases of metabolic alkalosis. For example, in the early phase of vomiting or nasogastric suctioning, a significant urinary bicarbonate wasting may occur. In such a situation, urinary sodium level is increased to balance the charge of the bicarbonate anion in urine. However, the urinary chloride level remains low, a very sensitive indicator of saline responsiveness. The usual causes of saline-responsive and saline-resistant metabolic alkaloses are shown in Table 2-1.

Further diagnostic investigation of the metabolic alkalemia produced the following values on spot urinary electrolyte readings:

Urinary sodium, 5 mEq/L
Urinary potassium, 40 mEq/L
Urinary chloride, 1 mEq/L

The low level of urinary chloride defines a saline-responsive metabolic alkalemia (the unmeasured urinary anion is probably bicarbonate).

Two distinct phases and events contribute to the metabolic alkalemia in the saline-responsive group. A loss of hydrogen ions causes a metabolic alkalemia triggered by sodium bicarbonate retention. In addition, a loss of plasma volume results from vomiting, nasogastric suction, diuretic use, or chloride-rich diarrhea.

The renal defense of this volume loss is the vigorous reabsorption of sodium. Since the kidney both manufactures bicarbonate in the proximal tubule (by the carbonic anhydrase mechanism) and filters an increased load of bicarbonate, reabsorbed sodium will be accompanied by bicarbonate as the reabsorbed anion. The volume loss and sodium bicarbonate reabsorption occur even though alkalemia develops, since volume maintenance is the kidney's primary role. Defense of volume will continue despite an increasing serum bicarbonate level and increasing serum pH.

Treatment of metabolic alkalemia and volume deficit. This patient should be treated symptomatically for the vomiting and receive intravenous normal saline with modest amounts of potassium chloride. This would decrease serum bicarbonate (because of a bicarbonate

---

Table 2-1. Causes of saline-responsive and saline-resistant metabolic alkalosis

Urinary chloride less than 10 mEq/L (saline-responsive)

Upper GI tract loss: vomiting, nasogastric suctioning

Lower GI tract loss: Chloride-rich diarrhea or villous adenoma

Posthypercapnia

Diuretic therapy

Urinary chloride greater than 20 mEq/L (saline-resistant)

Adrenal source: hyperaldosteronism, Cushing's disease and syndrome, iatrogenic (exogenous administration of glucocorticoid or mineralocorticoid)

Bartter's syndrome

Gitelman's syndrome

Liddle's syndrome

Ingestion of alkali

"Refeeding" alkalosis

Licorice ingestion

Table 2-2. Differential diagnosis of respiratory alkalosis

Endotoxemia (sepsis)

Chronic severe liver disease

CNS: Stroke, tumor or infection

Drugs that cause hyperventilation (eg, aspirin or other central nervous system stimulants)

Hyperthyroidism

Pulmonary causes: Hyperventilation/hypoxia, parenchymal lung disease or the effect of ventilators to decrease PCO_2

---

diuresis) and raise the serum potassium level, thereby correcting metabolic alkalemia and the volume deficit.

Differential diagnosis of respiratory alkalosis. The possible causes of respiratory alkalosis include underlying endotoxemia (sepsis), central nervous system disorders (Table 2-2), chronic severe liver disease, drug reactions that lead to hyperventilation, hyperthyroidism, and pulmonary disease with hypoxia-hyperventilation.

When respiratory alkalemia results from CNS dysfunction, drugs, or hypoxia, the source is usually evident clinically. If not, hidden causes — such as cirrhosis and endotoxemia — should be investigated thoroughly. Unexplained respiratory alkalemia is frequently related to sepsis. This clinical clue for endotoxemia may be the earliest indicator observable before septic shock ensues.

CASE 2-2. Patient with COPD and Diarrhea

Cases 2-2 and 2-3 illustrate how awareness of the presence of hypokalemia with an acid-base disorder significantly affects treatment.

A 65-year-old woman with chronic obstructive pulmonary disease (COPD) presents at a hospital emergency department with a 7 day history of diarrhea. She is confused and her breathing is labored. Her blood pressure is 100/60 mm Hg. Initial laboratory data include the following:

> Sodium, 137 mEq/L
> Potassium, 2.0 mEq/L
> Chloride, 111 mEq/L
> pH, 7.15
> PCO_2, 50 mm Hg
> Bicarbonate, 15 mEq/L

Use the five clinical rules to characterize the acid-base disorder (Table 1-1):

1. **Acidemia** is present (pH is less than 7.40).

2. The primary process is both **respiratory** (PCO_2 greater than 40) and **metabolic** (bicarbonate is decreased).

3. **Anion gap** is normal:

   $137 - (111 + 15) = 11$.

4. **Compensation.** This need not be calculated, since the coexistence of two acidemic disorders (metabolic and respiratory) makes the calculation for compensation moot.

5. **1:1 Relationship.** In a nonanion gap metabolic acidosis, the decline in bicarbonate should equal the increase in serum chloride. The bicarbonate level dropped to 15 mEq/L from 25 mEq/L (change of 10), and the chloride level increased to 111 mEq/L from 100 mEq/L (change of 11), demonstrating a relationship of almost 1:1, which confirms that there is no hidden metabolic alkalosis. Therefore, a third acid-base disturbance is absent.

Differential diagnosis of respiratory acidosis. Comparing the patient's current records to earlier ones often helps determine the primary process in a mixed acid-base situation. This patient's previous chart showed a pH of 7.34; PCO_2, 55 mm Hg; and bicarbonate, 32 mEq/L. These values are characteristic of a "pure" chronic respiratory acidemia in the setting of this patient's COPD (Table 2-3).

Differential diagnosis of metabolic acidemia. This patient's pH declined to 7.15 from 7.33 because a nonanion gap metabolic acidemia was superimposed on the chronic respiratory acidemia. The easiest approach to differential diagnosis of normal anion gap metabolic acidemia is a distinction between bicarbonate loss from a renal dysfunction (usually a tubular defect) and bicarbonate loss secondary to the gastrointestinal tract (loss of bicarbonate-rich fluids) (Table 2-4).

One approach to the differentiation of nonanion gap metabolic acidosis is measurement of urinary electrolytes. The normal kidney responds to GI-tract loss of bicarbonate (acidemia) by a compensatory increase in "titratable acidity" of urine. This can be indirectly measured by an apparent excess of negative charge —the so-called **urine delta gap**. The

Table 2-3. Major causes of respiratory acidemia

Pulmonary parenchymal disease such as COPD

Laryngospasm

Pleural disease

Impaired respiratory mechanics: sedation, muscular weakness, thoracic cage abnormality, or lesions of central respiratory center

Table 2-4. Causes of metabolic acidosis (nonanion gap)
Renal causes
Renal tubular acidosis, carbonic anhydrase inhibitors, acute or chronic renal failure, urinary tract obstruction, toluene inhalation, amphotericin B
GI tract causes
Bicarbonate-rich diarrhea, pancreatic fluid loss, ureteral diversions
Other causes
Posthypocapnic acidosis; ammonium, lysine, and arginine hydrochloride administration; sulfur toxicity

"unmeasured" positive ion responsible for the apparent excess of negative charges is ammonium (NH_4^+).

In this case, the patient's initial urine chemistries included:

> Urine pH, 5.00
> Urinary sodium, 10 mEq/L
> Urinary potassium, 30 mEq/L
> Urinary chloride, 100 mEq/L

The formula for the calculation of the urine delta gap is (sodium + potassium) – chloride. In this case, $(10 + 30) - 100 = -60$. The net urine change of -60 implies a substantial amount of urine acid (NH_4^+) excretion. This is consistent with a normal renal response to metabolic acidemia. Thus, this patient's diarrhea is the cause of the nonanion gap metabolic acidemia.

The gap in urine previously was called the urine anion gap. The utility of this concept, however, has extended to indirect measures of urinary bicarbonate in metabolic alkalosis. For example, urinary electrolytes in metabolic alkalosis — sodium, 10 mEq/L; potassium, 30 mEq/L; chloride, 1 mEq/L — and a urine pH of 7.5 have a gap of $(10 + 30) - 1 = 39$ "excess" positive charges that are balanced by urinary bicarbonate. Thus, urine delta gap is a more accurate name, encompassing as it does both "excess" positive and negative urine charges.

Note the patient's very low serum potassium concentration. The appropriate treatment of acidemia in a setting of severe hypokalemia is addressed in Case 2-3.

CASE 2-3. Progressive Symmetric Weakness with Near Respiratory Arrest

The acid-base and potassium-depletion status in this case is similar to that in Case 2-2, but with a very different cause.

A 16-year-old woman is admitted to the hospital with presumed Guillain-Barré syndrome. She has suffered progressive symmetric weakness resulting in near paralysis for the past week. Initial laboratory data include:

> Sodium, 136 mEq/L
> Potassium, 1.8 mEq/L
> Chloride, 114 mEq/L
> pH, 7.25
> PCO_2, 28 mm Hg
> Bicarbonate, 12 mEq/L

Use the five clinical rules to characterize the acid-base disorder (Table 1-1):

1. **Acidemia** is present (pH less than 7.40).

2. The primary process is **metabolic acidemia** (bicarbonate less than 25) and the PCO_2 is not high.

3. The **anion gap** is normal: $136 - (114 + 12) = 10$.

4. **Compensation.** As shown in Table 1-1, the compensation for metabolic acidosis is calculated thus: change in PCO_2 = 1.3 x decrease in bicarbonate. The bicarbonate is decreased by 13, so the PCO_2 should decrease to 23 (change in PCO_2 = 1.3 × 13 [25 − 12] = 17; 40 − 17 = 23).
   The initial PCO_2 is consistent with a mild superimposed respiratory acidosis. Therefore, compensation for the metabolic acidemia is not complete because the PCO_2 of 28 mm Hg is too high for normal compensation. A second disorder, respiratory acidosis, is present.

5. **1:1 Relationship.** This calculation suggests no underlying metabolic alkalosis: The chloride increases 14 mEq (to 114 from 100), and bicarbonate decreases 13 (to 12 from 25).

Once the electrolyte results became available, the profound weakness could be ascribed to severe potassium depletion rather than Guillain-Barré syndrome. During the next few minutes in the emergency department, the patient's respirations became increasingly labored, and repeat measurement of blood gases showed the following:

> Sodium, 136 mEq/L
> Potassium, 1.3 mEq/L
> Chloride, 113 mEq/L
> pH, 7.05
> PCO_2, 40 mm Hg

Bicarbonate, 12 mEq/L

The worsening of the acidosis in the hospital is solely due to a worsening of the respiratory acidosis (PCO_2 going from 28 to 40).

Treatment options. Since the initial moderately severe acidemia worsened, how should treatment proceed: intubation for the respiratory acidemia or IV administration of sodium bicarbonate for the metabolic process?

The important choice demonstrates that knowledge of a patient's potassium level is critical to the management of acid-base disorders. Bicarbonate administration would further lower the serum potassium level by driving potassium into cells. This aggravation of hypokalemia would cause additional muscle weakness and a potentially fatal respiratory arrest.

The use of the Five Rules shows the early development of respiratory acidemia (PCO_2 is 28, not 23). What could have been a "hidden" process was exposed by our follow-through with the calculations. The treatment of choice here — elective rather than emergent intubation — also was based on conclusions derived from the Five Rules. In case 2-2, the potassium reading of 2 mEq/L would have decreased if the pH of 7.15 had been increased by the administration of bicarbonate. The patient in Case 2-2 would then be very likely to retain more PCO_2 and potentially sustain a respiratory arrest.

The treatment of the patients' low potassium levels in both Cases 2-2 and 2-3 should consist of vigorous IV repletion with 20 to 30 mEq/L of potassium chloride per hour under cardiac-monitored guidance. When the potassium exceeds 3.2 mEq/L, the patient can be given bicarbonate gradually to correct the metabolic acidemia if the serum pH remains less than 7.10. If the pH is greater than 7.10, intravenous sodium bicarbonate is not necessary.

Differential diagnosis of metabolic acidemia. The approach we use to find the primary disturbance of nonanion gap metabolic acidemia is similar to that in Case 2-2: the urine pH and urine gap. This patient's initial spot urine test yielded these readings:

Urine pH, 7.00
Urinary sodium, 20 mEq/L
Urinary potassium, 30 mEq/L
Urinary chloride, 58 mEq/L

The urine gap is thus calculated: (Urine sodium + potassium) – chloride. The urine gap is (20 + 30) – 58 = – 8. The fact that there are only 8 excess negative charges is consistent with a subnormal acidification response to acidosis. This implicates the kidney as the source of the nonanion gap metabolic acidemia, and it eliminates other potential causes listed in Table 2-4. This presentation is most consistent with a distal renal tubular acidosis.

Case 2-4. Triple Acid-base Disorder

A 50-year-old man with a long history of ethanol abuse is hypotensive (100/50 mm Hg) when brought to the emergency department. The patient's friends say his recent drinking bout of several weeks' duration has been marked by anorexia punctuated by severe nausea and vomiting. Having run out of alcohol, he substituted antifreeze. He was found collapsed at home. Initial laboratory data include these findings:

> Sodium, 139 mEq/L
> Potassium, 6.5 mEq/L
> Chloride, 84 mEq/L
> pH, 6.86
> PCO_2, 81 mm Hg
> Bicarbonate, 16 mEq/L
> Glucose, 90 mg/dL
> Blood urea nitrogen (BUN), 48 mg/dL
> Ethanol, undetected

Use the five clinical rules to characterize the acid-base disorder:

1. **Severe acidemia** is present (pH less than 7.40).

2. The primary process is both **respiratory** (PCO_2 greater than 40) and **metabolic** (bicarbonate is decreased).

3. The **anion gap** is dramatically increased: $139 - (16 + 84) = 39$. This also indicates metabolic acidemia.

4. **Compensation.** This is moot because both acidemic processes are found in this patient.

5. **1:1 Relationship.** Bicarbonate is decreased ($25 - 16 = 9$), the anion gap is increased ($39 - 12 = 27$). The relative elevation of serum bicarbonate in this patient (the anion gap predicts a bicarbonate level near zero) suggests there is also a hidden metabolic alkalosis.

This patient has a **triple acid-base disorder** — anion gap metabolic acidemia, respiratory acidemia, and metabolic alkalosis. The patient's urinary electrolyte levels were:

> Urine pH, 5.00
> Urinary sodium, 1 mEq/L

Urinary potassium, 30 mEq/L
Urinary chloride, 8 mEq/L

These readings are consistent with saline-responsive metabolic alkalosis, probably secondary to vomiting.

Differential diagnosis of anion gap metabolic acidosis. A triple acid-base disorder, such as this man has, presents a significant diagnostic and treatment challenge. Intubation, required for cardiopulmonary arrest, corrected the acute respiratory acidemia and is the fastest way to partially correct the source acidemia.

Table 2-5 presents the differential diagnosis of anion gap metabolic acidosis. Both the patient's history and the profound elevation in anion gap suggest a diagnosis of antifreeze ingestion. If the history were not available, the serum osmol gap could provide a clue. The osmol gap is the difference between calculated serum osmolality ([2 × sodium] + [glucose/18] + [BUN/2.4] + [ethanol/4.6]) and the measured or actual serum osmolality. It normally is not greater than 10 to 15 mOsm/kg/ H_2O. For this patient, the following difference was observed:

$$
\begin{array}{ll}
\text{Sodium, } 139 \times 2 = & 278 \\
+\text{ Glucose, } 90/18 = & 5 \\
+\text{ BUN, } 48/2.4 \quad = & 20 \\
+\text{ Ethanol, } 0/4.6 \ = & 0 \\
\hline
& 303
\end{array}
$$

The patient's measured serum osmolality was 345.

The difference between the calculated and the measured osmolality (345 − 303 = 42) represents the presence of an **unmeasured active osmol.** In this case, without an increase in serum ethanol concentration, the serum osmol gap led to a diagnosis of ethylene glycol intoxication (oxalate being the unmeasured anion).

Importance of osmol gap in the treatment of metabolic acidemia. The combination of a high anion gap, metabolic acidemia, and a disparity in the osmol gap secondary to ethylene glycol ingestion led to a specific management strategy. After intubation, the patient was

---

Table 2-5. Causes of metabolic acidosis (anion gap)

Renal failure
Ketoacidosis (diabetic, alcohol-induced, gluconeogenic abnormality)
Lactic acidosis
Toxin ingestion: ethylene glycol, methanol, salicylates, paraldehyde

treated with volume expansion (normal saline for hypotension and metabolic alkalosis) and intravenous ethanol. Ethylene glycol and ethanol compete for the same enzyme — alcohol dehydrogenase — during liver metabolism. Ethanol competitively inhibits the conversion of ethylene glycol to oxalate and glyoxalate, which are toxic. Subsequent hemodialysis removed the ethylene glycol and its metabolites, and the serum anion gap and serum osmol gap decreased simultaneously with resolution of the acidemia.

Because of the patient's hyperkalemia, the ECG showed mildly peaked T-waves. Intubation to correct respiratory acidemia raised the serum pH to 7.15 from 6.86. The initial potassium concentration of 6.5 mEq/L decreased to 5.6. This occurred because potassium moved into cells, balancing the movement of hydrogen ions out of cells with the rise in pH. The ECG reverted to normal. Correction of acidemia is an effective tool for the treatment of hyperkalemia.

Note that at this point there are only two potential triple acid-base disturbances. This patient was found to have respiratory acidemia, metabolic acidemia, and metabolic alkalosis. The only other triple diagnostic possibility is the opposite respiratory category of alkalosis with both metabolic acid-base disturbances. Obviously, the differing components in triple acid-base disturbances can lead to a variable pH, which may be acidemic, alkalemic, or even normal under some circumstances.

Clinical highlights

To simplify interpretation of acid-base data, routinely follow these five rules: determine the pH status, assess whether the primary process is respiratory and/or metabolic, calculate the serum anion gap, check the degree of compensation, and find out whether there is a 1:1 relationship between anions in the blood.

Low levels of urinary chloride characterize saline-responsive metabolic alkalemia; high levels are associated with saline-resistant alkalemia.

Respiratory alkalemia resulting from CNS dysfunction, drugs, or hypoxia is usually straightforward. Unexplained respiratory alkalemia is frequently related to sepsis or severe liver disease.

Differentiation of nonanion gap metabolic acidosis is best done by measurement of urinary electrolytes through calculation of the urine delta gap.

In the presence of anion gap metabolic acidosis, measurement of the serum osmol gap — the difference between calculated and actual serum osmolality — can be helpful when the patient's clinical history is unclear.

Suggested Readings:

1. Goldstein MB, Bear R, Richardson RMA, et al. The urine anion gap: a clinically useful index of ammonium excretion. *Am J Med Sci.* 1986; 292:198-202.

2. Goldstein MB, Levin A. Insights derived from the urine in acid-base disturbances. *Am Kidney Found Lett.* 1989; 6:19-26.

3. Saxena R, Rutecki GW, Whittier FC. Enterovesical fistula presenting as life-threatening normal anion gap metabolic acidemia. *Am J Kidney Dis.* 1997; 30:131-133.

4. Schelling JR, Howard RL, Winter SD, et al. Increased osmolal gap in alcoholic ketoacidosis and lactic acidosis. *Ann Intern Med.* 1990; 113:580-582.

5. Porter GA. The treatment of ethylene glycol poisoning simplified. *N Engl J Med.* 1988; 319:109-110.

6. Ammar KA, Hecherling PS. Ethylene glycol poisoning with a normal anion gap caused by concurrent ethanol ingestion: importance of the osmol gap. *Am J Kidney Dis.* 1996; 27:130-133.

7. Leon M, Graeber C. Absence of high anion gap metabolic acidosis in severe ethylene glycol poisoning: a potential effect of simultaneous lithium carbonate ingestion. *Am J Kidney Dis.* 1994; 23:313-316.

3. Hypokalemia
Clinical Implications, Consequences, and Corrective Measures

Regulation of serum potassium concentrations within very narrow confines (3.5 to 5.2 mEq/L) is crucial to the maintenance of life. From the second-to-second discharge of cardiac pacemaker tissue that determines heart rhythm, to the force of diaphragmatic and accessory muscle contraction that is essential to ventilation, to the action potentials transmitting the million impulses in the CNS, the activity of numerous organ systems depends on the transcellular potassium gradient that establishes the resting membrane potential of electrical tissue.

In light of the lethal potential of an elevated or decreased potassium level, it makes sense that the body has developed a number of precise mechanisms to maintain potassium homeostasis. Despite these effective mechanisms, however, disturbances in potassium metabolism still account for a substantial portion of the electrolyte disorders seen in daily practice.

Potassium Homeostasis

Although potassium is distributed throughout the body, it is predominantly an intracellular cation (Table 3-1). The normal extracellular potassium concentration of 3.5 to 5.2 mEq/L is accompanied by an intracellular potassium concentration of 150 mEq/L. The total body potassium store averages about 50 mEq/kg of body weight; the serum potassium concentration represents only 2% of this total.

The large chemical gradient between the inside and outside of cell membranes favors the exit of intracellular potassium to the extracellular compartment. This movement (the so-called repolarization process) is responsible for establishing the resting membrane potential (inside negative to outside positive). The same ratio of extracellular to intracellular potassium also accounts for the function of voltage-dependent channels essential for electrical excitation and its coupling to muscle contraction.

Normal diets provide a potassium load of approximately 60 to 100 mEq/d. Approximately 90% is absorbed by the bowel. Zero potassium balance (ie, equal input and output) thus may require a urinary potassium excretion as high as 90 mEq/d.

Since 20 to 30 mEq/d of urinary potassium excretion is obligatory (potassium is exchanged for sodium during sodium reabsorption), an inadequate dietary intake may lead to potassium depletion within weeks to months. This explains why elderly persons can become hypokalemic when subsisting on a "tea and toast" diet containing less than 30 mEq/d of potassium: ongoing obligatory urinary potassium losses are not matched by an adequate potassium intake.

Certain "rapid" and "slow" modulators of potassium loads adjust the ratio of intracellular to extracellular potassium that permits normal membrane and electrical function. The rapid modulators — necessary following ingestion of a potassium load from potassium-rich foods (eg, meat) — efficiently translocate excess potassium from the extracellular to the intracellular compartment in minutes; they include insulin and catecholamines. Although acid-base homeostasis takes longer to translocate potassium intracellularly (more than 30 to 60 minutes), it usually is considered a rapid modulator as well.

The slow but also necessary regulators of potassium balance include aldosterone and intact renal function. These regulators increase urinary potassium excretion within hours.

If excess serum potassium is not actively pumped into cells, the altered extracellular-intracellular gradient will adversely affect repolarization and the resting membrane potential. The postprandial movement of large amounts of potassium from extracellular to intracellular compartments occurs through insulin-mediated activation of sodium/potassium-ATPase located on cell membranes (via an insulin-mediated decrease in intracellular sodium concentration). Catecholamines regulate serum potassium concentration by a mechanism similar to that of insulin (ie, a membrane ATPase activation that depends on cyclic AMP).

Table 3-1. Relative concentrations of some major extracellular and intracellular components

Component	Extracellular concentration (mEq/L)	Intracellular concentration (mEq/L)
Sodium	140	10
Potassium	4	150
Calcium	2.4	0.0001
Magnesium	1.4	58
Proteins (as buffers)	5*	40[†]

*Equivalent to 2g/dL.
†Equivalent to 16 g/dL.

Examining the link between acid-base homeostasis and potassium metabolism

Acid-base homeostasis is integral to potassium metabolism. In clinical practice, hypokalemia and acid-base disorders frequently coexist. For example, concurrent hypokalemia and metabolic alkalosis may suggest that both disturbances are related to vomiting. Conversely, hypokalemia with metabolic acidosis may indicate a common pathophysiologic mechanism, such as renal tubular acidosis or severe diarrhea.

Measures to correct acid-base disturbances may affect serum potassium levels. Systemic acidosis may increase extracellular potassium concentration, while metabolic alkalosis may decrease it. Significant acidosis with either a normal or a low serum potassium level may suggest a substantial and concomitant total body potassium deficit (ie, in patients with diabetic ketoacidosis). If acidosis is then corrected—with IV bicarbonate, for example—without potassium supplementation, the potassium concentration may decrease to dangerously low levels.

Metabolic acidosis with an accompanying anion gap shifts intracellular potassium to the extracellular compartment if the acid anion is a mineral (eg, sulfate or chlorride). Conversely, organic metabolic acidosis (eg, production of lactate or keto acids) does not raise extracellular potassium levels as much.

Mineral acid anions remain in the extracellular space, creating an outside to inside cell negativity that increases potassium movement down a gradient. Since lactate and keto acids enter cells, the charge gradient for potassium movement is absent in organic anion gap acidosis. When potassium movement to the extracellular compartment occurs in mineral acidoses, potassium concentration increases approximately 0.6 mEq/L for each 0.1 pH-unit decrease. Unfortunately, the shift varies considerably, from 0.2 to 1.7 mEq/L per 0.1 pH-unit change.

In non-anion gap acidoses, potassium wasting may occur and levels of potassium during acidosis may not be predicted with accuracy.

The increase in serum potassium concentration during respiratory acidosis is less than that during mineral metabolic acidosis with a potassium change of approximately 0.1 mEq/L for each 0.1 pH-unit change. Metabolic alkalosis decreases the potassium concentration approximately 0.3 mEq/L for each 0.1 pH-unit increase; the reduction associated with respiratory alkalosis is 0.25 mEq/L for each 0.1 pH-unit change. Again, these figures serve as estimates and may vary considerably.

Although one may not always be able to predict an exact rise or fall in the serum potassium level for each type of coexisting acid-base disturbance, an approximation may facilitate the treatment of hypokalemic patients. A decrease of 1 mEq/L in serum potassium concentration represents a total body loss of approximately 350 mEq of potassium.

Over longer periods, aldosterone and renal function modulate potassium excesses. Aldosterone increases the distal tubular secretion of potassium into the urine. As components of renal function, renal blood flow and glomerular filtration rate (GFR) also contribute to potassium excretion.

Another critical renal mechanism for potassium excretion is urinary flow rate; oliguria (less than 400 mL/d) may precipitate a fatal degree of potassium retention. Significant reductions in GFR (less than 10 mL/min/m^2) may also interfere with potassium excretion. Together, these facts explain why those patients with renal failure who maintain good urine output (more than 400 mL/d) often remain eukalemic until the GFR is drastically reduced (ie, to less than 10 mL/min/m^2).

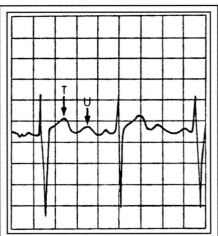

Figure 3-1. Note the u waves (arrow) with a prolonged QT-u interval in the ECG of the patient described in Case 3-1. The prolonged QT-u interval represents the extended time during which the ventricle is sensitive to premature electrical stimulation and thus ventricular tachycardia.

Effects of Hypokalemia

The untoward clinical consequences of potassium depletion predominantly affect the cardiovascular and neuromuscular systems. Both are a result of the associated hyperpolarization of electrical tissue.

For example, if the potassium concentration falls by 2 mEq/L, the absolute extracellular potassium concentrations are more profoundly affected than are intracellular concentrations. The extracellular-intracellular potassium gradient thus increases, hyperpolarizing the resting membrane potential. In addition, the presence of hypokalemia per se decreases membrane permeability to potassium. The resultant combination of effects prolongs action potentials, shortens refractory periods, and increases the incidence of spontaneous and early depolarization.

Cardiovascular system. For cardiac cells, the result of these alterations is a propensity for arrhythmias, particularly in persons who are taking digitalis. Since these effects may trigger ventricular fibrillation, they may be especially disastrous in patients with myocardial ischemia.

Hypokalemia-associated ECG findings include depressed ST segments, decreased T-wave amplitude, u waves, and a prolonged QT-u interval (Figure 3-1). The prolonged QT-u interval increases the likelihood of ventricular rhythm disturbances in patients with myocardial ischemia complicated by potassium depletion. This is especially true if other agents that prolong the QT-u interval (eg, quinidine) are administered (see Case 3-3).

Neuromuscular system. Hypokalemic hyperpolarization of skeletal muscle eventuates in varying degrees of muscle dysfunction (eg, weakness, myalgias, restless leg syndrome, cramps, and rhabdomyolysis) that may ultimately progress to respiratory muscle paralysis. In addition to exerting voltage effects on muscle, hypokalemia decreases glycogen storage and muscle blood flow; this further compromises contractile function.

Pancreas. The effects of potassium depletion on the pancreas — carbohydrate intolerance and decreased insulin release — are not life-threatening and will not be discussed further here.

Diagnosis and Management

Evaluating the hypokalemic patient for manifestations of associated target-organ dysfunction, such as arrhythmia and respiratory muscle weakness, helps gauge the severity of potassium depletion and determines the urgency of (and best approach to) treatment.

Thus, for hypokalemic patients with significant potassium depletion (levels less than 3 mEq/L), perform a focused physical examination to elicit any muscle weakness and obtain an ECG. The myopathy of hypokalemia is characterized by:

- Proximal rather than distal weakness (eg, difficulty in climbing stairs and combing hair is common)
- Preservation of reflexes
- Absence of sensory findings (including paresthesias)

These features help to distinguish hypokalemic myopathy from other neuropathies.

Mild hypokalemia (potassium concentration between 3.0 and 3.4 mEq/L) may be rapidly corrected by oral replacement; thus, the muscular examination and ECG may be unnecessary. Muscle dysfunction tends to be more severe with moderate or severe hypokalemia (2.9 mEq/L or less), but cardiac abnormalities may occur with lesser degrees of potassium depletion, especially if the patient has preexisting arrhythmias, ischemic heart disease, or is taking digitalis.

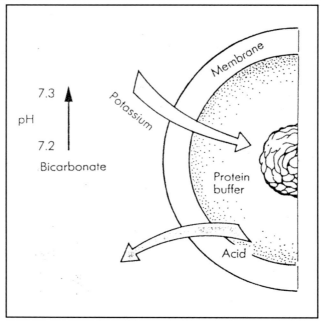

7.3

pH

7.2

Bicarbonate

Figure 3-2. Correction of acidemia and its impact on serum potassium. If the serum potassium level is already decreased during acidemia (see Case 3-1), correction of acidemia will shift buffered intracellular acid to the extracellular space and potassium will move to the intracellular space to maintain electroneutrality. The further decline in the potassium level may aggravate muscle weakness or arrhythmias. Some studies suggest that the drop in serum potassium level is a result of hemodilution and may not represent a shift.

The algorithm evaluating hypokalemia (see flowchart, "Evaluating hypokalemia") was designed to streamline your evaluation of potassium depletion. Categorizing the hypokalemic patient according to the presence or absence of an associated acid-base abnormality can facilitate the workup (Table 3-2). Table 3-3 provides some key points to help guide therapy.

Case 3-1. Hypokalemia with Metabolic Acidosis

Presentation. A 21-year-old woman presents to the emergency department with a complaint of symmetric muscle weakness (gradual worsening over 3 weeks; dramatic worsening during the prior 24 hours). She has no preceding medical history and is taking no licit or illicit medications. She specifically denies using diuretics or experiencing diarrhea.

The patient initially had difficulty in walking up stairs and rising from the bathtub. She is now barely able to lift her limbs against gravity.

Physical examination. Temperature: normal. Respirations: 24 breaths per minute and somewhat labored. Blood pressure: 110/60 mm Hg; pulse: 110 beats per minute and regular (supine). Blood pressure: 106/58 mm Hg; pulse: 116 beats per minute and regular (upright). The patient is alert, oriented, and anxious. Head, ears, eyes, nose, and throat: unremarkable. Heart, lungs, and abdomen: normal. Neurologic examination: symmetric but mildly decreased reflexes; sensory examination: normal. Muscle strength: markedly decreased in all the groups tested (proximal muscles more so than the distal muscles).

A tentative diagnosis of Guillain-Barre syndrome is made.

Laboratory findings.

Electrolyte levels:
      Sodium, 138 mEq/L
      Potassium, 2.4 mEq/L
      Chloride, 110 mEq/L
      Bicarbonate, 18 mEq/L.

      Glucose, 125 mg/dL
      BUN, 10 mg/dL
      Creatinine, 0.8 mg/dL
      WBC count, 8,300/mL with a normal differential.
      ECG, (Figure 3-1).

Since the patient is tachypneic and her serum bicarbonate concentration is abnormal, arterial blood gases are measured: pH 7.3; arterial oxygen tension (PaO_2), 86 mm Hg; arterial carbon dioxide tension ($PaCO_2$), 32 mm Hg; bicarbonate level, 18 mEq/L and normal compensation. The 1:1 ratio of Cl to HCO_3 is within normal variation.

The provisional diagnosis is then changed to hypokalemic muscle weakness of unknown cause with a simple metabolic acidemia.

Discussion. The association of hypokalemia with an acid-base disorder may help you identify the cause of potassium depletion. In addition to profound potassium depletion, this patient has metabolic acidemia.

Substantial losses of potassium and bicarbonate may occur through two major sites: the GI tract (via severe diarrhea or excessive laxative use) and the kidney (via renal tubular acidosis).

GI losses. Intestinal fluid is rich in potassium and bicarbonate. In patients with severe diarrhea, for example, hypokalemia with concurrent non-anion gap acidemia develops in response to the simultaneous loss of potassium and bicarbonate from the stool. The kidney compensates for these electrolyte losses through two mechanisms:

- Reabsorption of potassium from the filtrate
- Increased urinary acid excretion through the generation of ammonia, which then becomes ammonium in the tubular lumen. This is called titratable acidity.

Measurement of urinary electrolyte levels can help establish whether the renal response to gut loss of potassium and bicarbonate is intact, thereby implicating the stool as the site for potassium depletion and the cause of the acidemia. Thus, we provide sample spot urine electrolytes:

Sodium, 12 mEq/L
Potassium, 15 mEq/L
Chloride, 60 mEq/L; pH 5.5.

Note that urinary electrolyte analysis does not routinely include the bicarbonate concentration. Nonetheless, a so-called urine gap (or delta gap) may be calculated; it represents the difference between positive and negative charges. Like serum, urine always contains an equal number of positive and negative ions.

Calculation from this spot sample reveals 55 "unmeasured" positive charges ($[12\ Na^+ + 18\ K^+] + - 85\ Cl^- = -55$). (In essence, the 55 "excess" negative charges must be balanced by an unmeasured cation.) In the presence of systemic acidemia, the unmeasured positive charges represent ammonium as titratable acidity; normally, ammonium is generated and excreted by the kidney to compensate for the excess acid in the plasma.

Hypokalemia with a non-anion gap acidemia and urinary excretion of titratable acid (ammonium and low pH) is diagnostic of gut loss of potassium and bicarbonate. These spot urine values suggest that diarrhea or laxative abuse is causing hypokalemia and acidemia in the presence of a normal renal response to acidemia. Upon further questioning this patient admitted to surreptitious laxative abuse.

Kidney losses. On the other hand, the following sample spot urine values would incriminate the kidney as the source of both the potassium depletion and acidemia: sodium, 22 mEq/L; potassium, 35 mEq/L; chloride, 57 mEq/L; pH 7. These values would be consistent with distal renal tubular acidosis. The sum of the electrolyte charges shows neither a net secretion of ammonium nor a delta gap consistent with a renal defect in acid secretion ($[22\ Na^+ + 35\ K^+] + - 57Cl^- = 0$).

This is further corroborated by finding neutral rather than acidic urine in a patient with systemic acidosis: the kidney's normal response to systemic acidosis is absent in a patient with hypokalemia and acidemia resulting from renal tubular acidosis.

Table 3-2. Differential diagnosis of hypokalemia*

Type of hypokalemia	Possible causes
Secondary to potassium redistribution	Intracellular potassium shift in response to alkalemia or correction of acidemia; β-adrenergic agonists; insulin; unusual precipitants (eg, barium poisoning, RBC uptake of potassium during vitamin B_{12} therapy for macrocytic anemia)
Secondary to GI loss of potassium†	Diarrhea; vomiting or nasogastric suction; other GI fluid losses (eg, those associated with a villous adenoma)
Secondary to renal potassium wasting	Renal tubular acidosis; drugs (usually diuretics); mineralocorticoid excess; hypomagnesemia
Secondary to diet	Inadequate intake (eg, in elderly or alcoholic patients)
Secondary to rare disorders	Periodic paralysis (shift of potassium into muscle cells)

*Should all the listed causes be ruled out, consider the possibility of spurious hypokalemia. However, spurious hypokalemia is usually accompanied by a dramatically elevated WBC count (>100,000/µl), as may be seen in leukemia.

†May be associated with alkalemia secondary to upper GI tract loss or acidemia secondary to lower GI tract loss.

Table 3-3. Managing hypokalemia: a few basics

- To correct potassium depletion associated with significant muscle weakness or arrhythmia, use IV potassium chloride (10-30 mEq/h). Keep the patient in a monitored bed and have electrolyte levels checked frequently —overshooting the potassium level can be dangerous.

- To correct less severe potassium depletion, use oral potassium chloride (sustained-release preparations are acceptable) or IV potassium chloride (5-10 mEq/L).*

- Patient monitoring is suggested whenever the rate of IV potassium chloride administration exceeds 10 mEq/h.

- Correction of acidosis may shift extracellular (serum) potassium into the intracellular compartment. Thus, low serum potassium levels may decline even further as acidosis is corrected.

*Be cautious when using both oral sustained-release and IV potassium chloride, since an overshoot is possible.

Therapy. The approach depends on whether hypokalemic target-organ dysfunction is present and on the type of associated acid-base disturbance. This patient's ECG shows u waves but no other arrhythmia or evidence of ischemia, and she is not taking digitalis. She does, however, have profound muscle weakness on the neurologic examination. Decreased respiratory muscle strength may also lead to atelectasis and a ventilation-perfusion mismatch (PaO_2 of 86 mm Hg).

Additional worsening of this patient's muscle weakness could precipitate the development of further respiratory muscle compromise. Consequently, it is critical to consider her acid-base status not only during the diagnostic workup but also during treatment for hypokalemia.

For example, if the patient is given IV bicarbonate to raise her serum pH, her potassium concentration would decline further (Figure 3-2). Initial therapy must therefore focus primarily on correcting the low potassium level. IV potassium chloride (up to a rate of 20 to 30 mEq/h), administered with frequent electrolyte monitoring (at least every 2 hours), is recommended.

The fall in blood pressure associated with upright posture is consistent with the presence of concomitant volume contraction. This finding suggests the need for coadministration of normal saline (approximately 1 to 2 L over the first 12 hours).

Rapid and excessive saline expansion results in a kaliuresis (reabsorption of sodium by the tubules is coupled with potassium excretion) and may aggravate potassium depletion. Since it is impossible to predict the patient's exact potassium deficit, treatment must be carefully adjusted to normalize the serum and total body potassium concentrations.

Only after the potassium deficit and volume contraction are corrected should the acidemia be addressed. If diarrhea is causing the potassium depletion and acidemia, measures to relieve it will correct both disturbances. Renal loss of potassium and hydrogen attributable to renal tubular acidosis requires long-term therapy with divided oral doses of sodium bicarbonate (1 mEq/kg/d).

Laxative abuse is a definite consideration in any patient with unexplained hypokalemia, non-anion gap metabolic acidemia, and increased urinary ammonium excretion. Often, however, the patient will adamantly deny any such abuse.

Case 3-2. Hypokalemia with Metabolic Alkalosis

Presentation. A 42-year-old man with a history of peptic ulcer disease has been vomiting (without blood) for 2 weeks. Endoscopy had demonstrated an ulcer 2 years earlier, at which time treatment with H_2

blockers was started. Although *H. pylori* was present on biopsy, the patient did not complete his prescribed regimen and was lost to follow-up. Postprandial pain had recurred for 4 to 6 months before the recent episodes.

Physical examination. Blood pressure: 106/88 mm Hg; pulse: 98 beats per minute (supine). Blood pressure: 100/80 mm Hg; pulse: 116 beats per minute (upright). Remainder of the examination: normal, except for the presence of mild epigastric tenderness on palpation. Muscle strength: symmetric and normal.

Laboratory findings.

Serum electrolyte levels
    Sodium, 132 mEq/L
    Potassium, 2.9 mEq/L
    Chloride, 96 mEq/L
    Bicarbonate, 36 mEq/L.
ECG: sinus tachycardia only.
Urinary electrolyte levels:
    Sodium, 20 mEq/L
    Potassium, 34 mEq/L
    Chloride, 1 mEq/L
Urinary pH: 7.5.

Discussion. Here hypokalemia is associated with vomiting and an elevated serum bicarbonate level (normal range, 24 to 26 mEq/L). This combination of electrolytes (combined potassium deficit and bicarbonate surplus) suggests a metabolic alkalosis. Furthermore, the low spot urinary chloride level is consistent with vomiting and volume depletion, or a so-called saline-responsive metabolic alkalosis accompanied by potassium depletion. The excess positive urine charge or gap ([20 Na^+ + 34 K^+] −1 Cl^- = 53) is attributable to unmeasured bicarbonaturia (ie, 53 "excess" positive charges are present).

From a treatment perspective, the patient has no target-organ disturbances from hypokalemia — muscle strength and the ECG are normal. Arterial blood gas measurements demonstrate a metabolic alkalemia (pH 7.54).

Therapy. Normal saline will correct the volume disturbance and lower the bicarbonate level and pH toward normal. Although the decrease in pH will raise the serum potassium concentration, the potassium depletion is enough that IV potassium chloride (approximately 20 mEq/h), together with at least 4 to 6 L of normal saline over the first 24 hours, is recommended. As in Case 3-1, therapy must be adjusted for the particular patient. The vigorous saline repletion in this patient

How hypokalemia affects the extracellular-intracellular potassium ratio

The extracellular fluid space in a 70-kg adult is 14 L (20% of 70 kg). A normal serum potassium level of 4 mEq/L would amount to a total of 56 mEq (4×14) of potassium.

At the same time, the intracellular fluid space is approximately 21 L. It contains 150 mEq/L of potassium, which represents a total of 3,150 mEq of potassium (21×150; Figure).

A decline in the serum potassium level from 4 to 2 mEq/L would correspond to a total body loss of potassium of approximately 700 mEq (350 mEq for every 1 mEq/L decline). The serum potassium level of 2 mEq/L in the extracellular space would represent a total body loss of potassium of 28 mEq (2×14). The remaining potassium loss (700 - 28 = 672 mEq/L) would come from the intracellular space.

The percentage change for each cellular fluid space would be:
Extracellular: 28/56 = 50%
Intracellular: 672/3,150 = 21%

presumes normal cardiovascular function.

The low spot urinary chloride concentration is accompanied by a relatively low urinary sodium level. If vomiting had been present for less than 72 hours, the urinary chloride level would still be low but the urinary sodium level may be above 20 mEq/L. Before renal tubular compensation for the loss of volume (increased sodium bicarbonate reabsorption) results, a bicarbonate diuresis accompanied by a loss of sodium and potassium occurs. Only those low-chloride alkaloses caused by early vomiting or nasogastric suction (for less than 72 hours) are associated with the increased urinary sodium secretion necessitated by bicarbonate diuresis.

Subsequent workup reveals that an obstructing channel ulcer is responsible for the patient's vomiting. Correcting the obstruction will normalize and maintain the potassium level and acid-base status. *H. pylori* treatment is completed later and the bacterium is eradicated.

Figure 3-4 shows another category of potassium depletion and metabolic alkalosis: that marked by a high urinary chloride concentration. Affected patients (unlike those who are saline-responsive) are not volume-depleted. The alkalemia and potassium depletion associated with elevated urinary chloride levels occur when there is an excess of a mineralocorticoid such as aldosterone (secondary to tumor, hyperplasia, or high renin states); corticosteroids (secondary to Cushing's disease or syndrome); or exogenous mineralocorticoids (secondary to licorice ingestion) (Table 2-1).

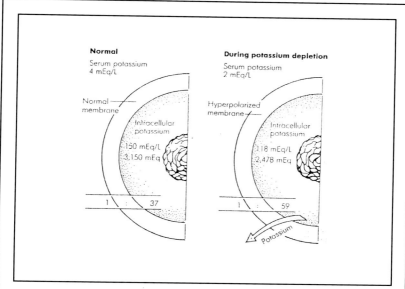

Figure 3-3. The ratio of extracellular to intracellular potassium under normal conditions and during potassium depletion. A decline in potassium concentration to 2 mEq/L raises the intracellular to extracellular (transcellular) potassium concentration gradient from 37:1 to 59:1. This increase necessitates greater potassium movement out of cells and thus is associated with hyperpolarization of the resting membrane potential. The Nernst equation can be used to approximate the resting cellular transmembrane potential, which is equal to:

$$-61 \log \frac{\text{Intracellular potassium concentration}}{\text{Extracellular potassium concentration}}$$

Licorice contains glycyrrhizic acid, which inhibits 11b-hydroxysteroid dehydrogenase, the enzyme that converts cortisol to cortisone. Cortisol activates renal mineralocorticoid receptors, and its excess from licorice ingestion can lead to potassium wasting, alkalosis, and hypertension. However, the amount of licorice that must be ingested for this to occur is excessive, making these complications rare.

Comment. Cases 3-1 and 3-2 illustrate how simultaneously considering potassium depletion and acid-base status makes sense for both diagnosis and treatment. Potassium depletion and non-anion gap acidemia occur only via lower gut loss of fluid and renal loss of potassium and bicarbonate. Potassium depletion with alkalemia may coexist with low or high urinary levels of chloride.

Evaluating hypokalemia

Measurement of serum electrolyte levels reveals potassium depletion (serum potassium level below 3.5 mEq/L).*

↓

Assess acid-base status (measure serum bicarbonate level; measure arterial blood gases if bicarbonate level is abnormal.

Metabolic acidosis or acidema (often—but not always—unaccompanied by an elevated *serum* anion gap)

Consider possible causes:

↓

• Lower GI tract loss of potassium and bicarbonate via diarrhea or laxative abuse. Urinary electrolyte levels consistent with "hidden" ammonium excretion or a so-called delta gap.
• Renal loss of potassium and bicarbonate attributable to renal tubular acidosis or use of carbonic anhydrase inhibitors. Urinary electrolyte levels without the increased "hidden" positive ammonium charges (no generation of ammonium by kidney); urinary pH above 6 (by dipstick) in renal tubular acidosis despite the acidosis.
• Acidosis accompanied by an elevated serum anion gap (eg, diabetic ketoacidosis) possibly associated with simultaneous potassium depletion and metabolic acidosis.

Normal acid-base status

↓

Consider possible causes:

↓

• Renal loss of magnesium attributable to medications (eg, cisplatin, aminoglycosides,).
• Hypokalemia attributable to periodic paralysis.
• Renal loss of potassium attributable to diuretics.†
• Poor dietary intake of potassium.

Metabolic alkalosis or alkalemia

↓

Consider possible causes:

↓

• Upper GI tract loss of potassium and hydrochloride via vomiting or nasogastric suction. (Low spot urinary chloride levels.)
• Renal loss of potassium attributable to diuretics.† (Volume depletion makes patients saline-responsive.)
• Mineralocorticoid excess possibly accompanied by hypertension. (High urinary chloride level.)

*In the absence of the leukocytosis (>100,000/mL) seen in leukemia, whereby WBCs may take up potassium on standing, this level of potassium depletion can lead to an in vitro (but not an in vivo) hypokalemia.

†Diuretic-related hypokalemia may be associated with alkalosis or may be present in the absence of an acid-base disorder.

When planning treatment, take into account the effect of the systemic pH change during or after interventions directed at regulating potassium movement into or out of cells. Correcting acidemia lowers the potassium level further and can cause serious consequences if potassium depletion already exists.

CASE 3-3. Hypokalemia with Normal Acid-base Status

Presentation. A 72-year-old man presents with CHF. The history reveals two previous MIs complicated by ischemic cardiomyopathy and an ejection fraction of 30%. His current medication regimen consists of digoxin, 0.25 mg/d (plasma levels are therapeutic); furosemide, 40 mg/d; captopril, 25 mg tid; and one adult-strength aspirin daily. He experienced shortness of breath and paroxysmal nocturnal dyspnea with chest pain 24 hours before admission.

Physical findings. Blood pressure: 160/70 mm Hg; pulse: 110 beats per minute (upright). Blood pressure: 165/86 mm Hg; pulse: 110 beats per minute (supine). Respirations: 24 breaths per minute and labored. Temperature: normal. Chest: rales throughout both lower lung fields. Vascular: jugular venous distention to the angle of the jaw at 30 degrees. Cardiac: left ventricular hypertrophy by palpation, an S_4 and S_3, ectopy (premature ventricular contractions), and a holosystolic (2/6) murmur that transmits to the left axilla. Lower extremities: edema (4+). Neuromuscular: normal. ECG findings: see Figure 3-5.

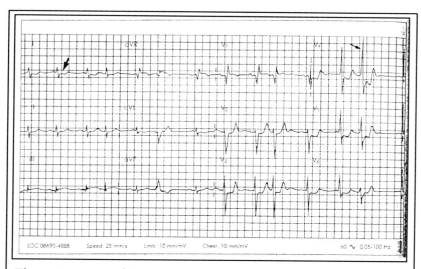

Figure 3-5. ECG of the patient described in Case 3-3 reveals ectopic beats (premature ventricular complexes; small arrow) and abnormal ST segments (large arrow) attributable to ischemia.

Laboratory findings.

Electrolyte levels
     Sodium, 130 mEq/L
     Potassium, 3mEq/L
     Chloride, 102 mEq/L
     Bicarbonate, 23 mEq/L.
BUN, 32 mg/dL
Creatinine, 1.7 mg/dL.
Arterial blood gas measurements
     PaO_2, 80 mm Hg
     $PaCO_2$, 30 mm Hg
     Bicarbonate, 24 mEq/L
     pH 7.44.
     Magnesium, 1.2 mEq/L.

Discussion. This patient has hypokalemia with ventricular ectopy and is taking digitalis; neither acidosis nor alkalosis is present. The decreased potassium level may be related to poor intake and/or the diuretic's effect on potassium and magnesium levels.

When potassium depletion is unaccompanied by an acid-base disorder, a number of other considerations must be taken into account. In patients who have cardiac disease, the most important of these is whether they have a magnesium deficiency.

This patient's magnesium level was low (normal, 1.4 to 1.8 mEq/L). Diuretics waste potassium and magnesium in the urine, and a deficiency of both cations increases the likelihood of a ventricular rhythm disturbance being present.

Treatment of CHF is required along with repletion of magnesium and potassium levels under cardiac monitoring. Appropriate parenteral regimens for magnesium depletion are:

- 2 g of magnesium chloride in 100 mL of normal saline over 30 to 60 minutes, with a follow-up serum magnesium measurement and further doses of magnesium as necessary
- 4 mL of 50% magnesium sulfate in 100 to 200 mL of dextrose 5% in water over 30 minutes, followed by 10 mL in 1 L of dextrose 5% in water over 24 hours

Oral magnesium replacement may be associated with diarrhea. In this patient, a regimen for potassium repletion resembling Case 2 (e.g., averaging 10 to 20 mEq/h IV) is recommended. Reevaluate electrolyte levels every 2 to 4 hours over the first 12 hours to prevent overshooting magnesium and potassium concentrations, a potentially lethal complication.

Obviously, general medical considerations also include whether the patient has sustained a recent non-Q wave MI. The presence of an acute infarct makes the management of potassium depletion more critical, since ventricular tachycardia-fibrillation is possible.

Suggested Reading

1. Braden GL, von Deyer PT, Germain MJ et al. Ritodrine- and terbutaline-induced hypokalemia in preterm labor: mechanisms and consequences. *Kid Int.* 1997; 51:1867-1875.

2. Donowitz M, Kokke FT, Saidi R. Evaluation of patients with chronic diarrhea. *N Engl J Med.* 1995; 332:725-729.

3. Gennari FS. Hypokalemia. *N Engl J Med.* 1998; 339:451-458.

4. Kamel KS, Halperin ML, Faber MD, et al. Disorders of potassium balance. In: Brenner BM, ed. *The Kidney.* 5th ed. Philadelphia: WB Saunders; 1996 5:999-1037.

5. Kobrin SM. Magnesium deficiency. *Semin Nephrol.* 1990;10:525-535.

6. Weiner ID, Wingo CS. Hypokalemia — Consequences, causes, and correction. *J Am Soc Nephrol.* 1997; 8:1179-1188.

4. Hyperkalemia
How to Identify—and Correct—the Underlying Cause

Unless serum potassium concentrations are maintained within very narrow limits (3.5 to 5.2 mEq/L), contractile and excitable tissues cannot function normally. When potassium homeostasis goes awry, the result may be profound muscle weakness and potentially fatal cardiac rhythm disturbances.

Effects of Hyperkalemia

Intracellular-extracellular potassium movement. As the extracellular potassium level increases, the intracellular-extracellular transmembrane gradient for potassium movement declines. The diminished potassium movement decreases the resting membrane potential (the converse of hypokalemia-related membrane hyperpolarization); thus depolarizing the membrane and interfering with repolarization. The slowed propagation and conduction of action potentials may also adversely affect skeletal muscle and lead to flaccid paralysis.

ECG findings. Always include an ECG when evaluating a hyperkalemic patient for target-organ dysfunction. Unfortunately, the correlation between the presence of hyperkalemia and the ECG findings is not completely reliable. Nonetheless, the absolute level of serum potassium combined with an ECG is still the best measure of hyperkalemic target-organ dysfunction.

The progression of ECG abnormalities that may occur during hyperkalemia may be seen best on leads V_2, V_3, and V_4 (Figure 4-2):

- Tall peaked T waves (these usually occur at potassium concentrations between 5.5 and 6.5 mEq/L)

- Decreased amplitude and eventual absence of the P wave (at potassium levels between 7 and 8 mEq/L)

- QRS widening caused by progressive intraventricular conduction abnormalities that evolve into a sine wave pattern, ventricular tachycardia, and ventricular fibrillation (usually at potassium levels above 7 mEq/L; however, this pattern may occur at lower potassium levels as well).

Figure 4-1. Algorithm for Evaluating hyperkalemia

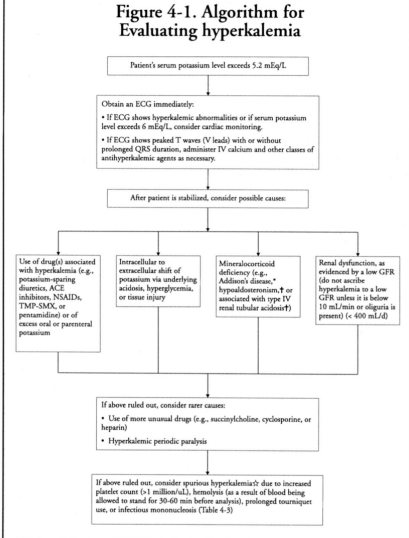

Patient's serum potassium level exceeds 5.2 mEq/L

Obtain an ECG immediately:

• If ECG shows hyperkalemic abnormalities or if serum potassium level exceeds 6 mEq/L, consider cardiac monitoring.

• If ECG shows peaked T waves (V leads) with or without prolonged QRS duration, administer IV calcium and other classes of antihyperkalemic agents as necessary.

After patient is stabilized, consider possible causes:

Use of drug(s) associated with hyperkalemia (e.g., potassium-sparing diuretics, ACE inhibitors, NSAIDs, TMP-SMX, or pentamidine) or of excess oral or parenteral potassium	Intracellular to extracellular shift of potassium via underlying acidosis, hyperglycemia, or tissue injury	Mineralocorticoid deficiency (e.g., Addison's disease,* hypoaldosteronism,† or associated with type IV renal tubular acidosis†)	Renal dysfunction, as evidenced by a low GFR (do not ascribe hyperkalemia to a low GFR unless it is below 10 mL/min or oliguria is present) (< 400 mL/d)

If above ruled out, consider rarer causes:

• Use of more unusual drugs (e.g., succinylcholine, cyclosporine, or heparin)

• Hyperkalemic periodic paralysis

If above ruled out, consider spurious hyperkalemia☆ due to increased platelet count (>1 million/uL), hemolysis (as a result of blood being allowed to stand for 30-60 min before analysis), prolonged tourniquet use, or infectious mononucleosis (Table 4-3)

GFR, glomerular filtration rate; TMP-SMX, trimethoprim-sulfamethoxazole.

*Look for decreased blood pressure, pigmentation, and hyponatremia along with an elevated serum potassium level.

†Particularly likely in diabetic patients.

☆ Although many experts consider the possibility of spurious hyperkalemia earlier in the evaluation, we believe that initial consideration of the ECG findings and the potential causes of "real" hyperkalemia constitutes a safer approach.

Gradual elevations in potassium concentration may follow this classic ECG evolution. More sudden elevations of potassium, however, may not follow the typical pattern and may eventuate in ventricular fibrillation without warning. Thus, the blood level of potassium is important even when the ECG is normal. Conversely, a patient whose ECG is abnormal despite a minimally elevated potassium level merits appropriate treatment.

Management Principles

Sound management of hyperkalemia depends on determining which therapies will effectively lower the potassium level and how urgently treatment is needed (the latter is based on the serum potassium level and the ECG conduction abnormalities).

Three treatment options are available:

- IV calcium (a membrane stabilizer)

- Agents that shift excess extracellular potassium into cells

- Agents and methods that remove potassium from the body.

Each exerts different effects on elevated potassium levels.

IV calcium. Administered as a gluconate or chloride salt, IV calcium is a direct but temporary antagonist to the effects of hyperkale-

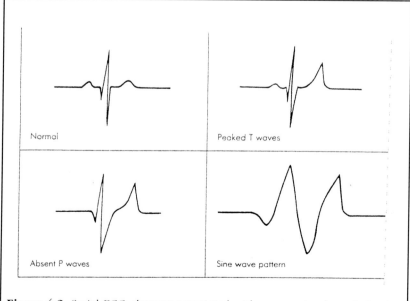

Figure 4-2. Serial ECG changes associated with progressive hyperkalemia.

mia on the cardiac conduction system. It elevates the threshold membrane potential but does not shift excess potassium into cells or remove potassium from the body.

When hyperkalemic cardiac conduction abnormalities are more severe (eg, when t waves are markedly peaked or the QRS widened), IV calcium is the initial treatment of choice. Nonetheless, always supplement IV calcium with additional, more definitive therapy; otherwise, the life-threatening rhythm disturbances will return within an hour or two.

Shifting agents. Insulin, sodium bicarbonate, and β-agonists shift excess extracellular potassium into cells. Insulin-mediated movement of potassium into cells is accompanied by a similar movement of glucose. Thus, if 50% glucose and insulin are given IV, potassium will enter the intracellular compartment concurrently with cellular glucose uptake. In general, administer insulin and IV glucose together to avoid inducing hypoglycemia; such coadministration is unnecessary when diabetes-related hyperglycemia already exists.

Sodium bicarbonate produces alkalemia in the extracellular compartment; this promotes a shift of acid from intracellular to extracellular locations. The movement of acid from the intracellular to extracellular compartment to buffer the bicarbonate necessitates the transfer of extracellular potassium to the intracellular compartment to maintain electroneutrality.

β-agonist-induced stimulation of β-adrenergic receptors also shifts extracellular potassium into cells. The effect is mediated by activation of cyclic AMP and the sodium-potassium pump. In addition, certain β-agonists (eg, albuterol) directly stimulate β-receptors in the pancreas, thereby increasing insulin levels. These two effects appear to be additive in that insulin activates the sodium-potassium pump further through a different method of cyclic AMP stimulation.

Albuterol has been studied in patients with chronic renal failure — a group that is particularly prone to hyperkalemia. When given IV or by inhalation, albuterol may facilitate efforts to shift potassium intracellularly during hyperkalemia.

The underlying problem with all these agents is that they shift excess extracellular potassium only temporarily and do not remove it from the body. If such an agent is the sole therapy, potassium levels will again rise.

Removal agents and methods. Sodium polystyrene sulfonate, an ion exchange resin, removes potassium from the body by exchanging it for sodium. Mixing the resin with sorbitol can make it palatable — although not appetizing — and is important to ward off the constipation caused by the resin itself. It may be administered orally or by rectal retention enemas.

The oral route requires a functional GI tract and poses a risk of aspiration in patients with altered mentation. Doses administered rectally may not be retained long enough to be effective and thus may not remove sufficient potassium to prevent serious arrhythmias.

Because ion exchange resin takes hours to remove significant amounts of potassium from the body, use another treatment option (eg, IV calcium) in emergent situations.

Dialysis is the most definitive way to remove potassium permanently. Large amounts of potassium may be removed if the potassium concentration of the hemodialysate is kept at 2 mEq/L or less. Treatment with a **potassium-wasting diuretic**, such as furosemide or a thiazide, is a mainstay of therapy in hyperkalemic patients with preserved renal function. Since volume loss accompanies diuretic-induced potassium wasting, give IV fluids (dextrose 5% in normal or half-normal saline) to maintain fluid volume.

We have designed an Algorithm (Figure 4-1) to simplify the work-up of hyperkalemic patients. In addition, we have summarized the differential diagnosis of and treatment options for hyperkalemia (Tables 4-1 and 4-2).

CASE 4-1. Diabetes-related Hyperkalemia

A 32-year-old woman has had insulin-dependent diabetes mellitus for 18 years. Background diabetic retinopathy was discovered about 3 years ago, and she recently underwent laser treatments for retinal hemorrhages.

Significant proteinuria (2.1 g in 24 hours) was subsequently found a year later. The protein loss was associated with an elevated creatinine level, which has risen from 0.9 to 2 mg/dL over the last 18 months.

Three months ago, the patient came in for an office visit. Her blood pressure was 150/98 mm Hg. Electrolyte levels were as follows:

> Sodium, 138 mEq/L
> Potassium, 4.8 mEq/L
> Chloride, 106 mEq/L
> Bicarbonate, 20 mEq/L.

In light of recent studies suggesting the effectiveness of ACE

Table 4-1. Differential diagnosis of hyperkalemia	
Cause	**Mechanisms**
Redistribution of potassium from intracellular to extracellular compartments	Release of intracellular potassium during tissue injury (eg, rhabdomyolysis; see Case 4-2); intravascular hemolysis (see Case 4-2); diabetes-related hypertonicity
Excess potassium from increased intake or decreased excretion	Medications, such as triamterene, pentamidine, amiloride, ACE inhibitors, and NSAIDs (see Cases 4-1 and 4-3); excess oral or IV potassium loading; salt substitutes, particularly in the presence of chronic renal insufficiency (see Case 4-1); diet
Hormonal abnormalities	Decreased aldosterone synthesis or release (eg, type IV renal tubular acidosis, ACE inhibitors; see Case 4-1); Addison's disease (see Case 4-3)
Renal failure with or without oliguria	Decreased urinary and glomerular filtration rates
Pseudo- or spurious hyperkalemia	Elevated platelet counts; allowing blood samples to stand for 30 to 60 minutes before being analyzed; infectious mononucleosis

inhibitors in diabetic patients with renal disease, her physician prescribed captopril (25 mg twice a day). Spironolactone (25 mg twice a day) was also given to correct coexistent 2+ peripheral edema.

After 2 weeks on this regimen, the patient's blood pressure has fallen to 130/88 mm Hg, and she is asymptomatic. ECG findings are normal. Electrolyte levels:

> Sodium, 136 mEq/L
> Potassium, 5.8 mEq/L
> Chloride, 108 mEq/L
> Bicarbonate, 18 mEq/L

Differential diagnosis. In primary care, persons with diabetes and mild renal insufficiency (like the patient in this case history) are the ones who most often have hyperkalemia. Such persons are prone to the development of life-threatening hyperkalemia from a number of mechanisms.

Hypoaldosteronism. Aldosterone plays an important role in the excretion of potassium. Renal excretion of potassium depends on urinary flow rates (400 mL/d or less interferes with potassium excretion); adequate glomerular filtration rate ([GFR]; potassium excretion is compromised at GFRs of less than 10 mL/min); and aldosterone (which increases distal tubular potassium excretion).

For unknown reasons, diabetes with early nephropathy is frequently associated with hypoaldosteronism and type IV renal tubular acidosis. This patient's renal function is more than adequate to excrete excess potassium: her urinary volume is adequate, and the serum creatinine is only 2mg/dL. The disturbed potassium excretion most likely results from a low aldosterone concentration that does not increase appropriately in response to hyperkalemia.

Medications. NSAIDs, as well as many drugs used for treating diabetic patients with renal insufficiency (eg, **ACE inhibitors** and **potassium-sparing diuretics,** such as spironolactone), further decrease the level of aldosterone and its target-organ effects.

Both prescription and OTC NSAIDs may further reduce GFRs and aldosterone levels in diabetic patients and exacerbate the defective potassium excretion. Although NSAIDs do not produce significant renal effects in healthy patients, they may cause a number of problems in patients who are elderly or who have renal disease.

NSAIDs may reduce renal blood flow and the GFR thus leading to oliguria. They may also decrease aldosterone release by unclear mechanisms. In diabetic patients, the effects of oliguria and a further decline in aldosterone levels can precipitate life-threatening hyperkalemia.

ACE converts angiotensin I to angiotensin II, which stimulates the adrenal cortex to release aldosterone. ACE inhibitors thus have the potential to interfere with potassium excretion, especially in those diabetic patients whose baseline aldosterone level may be perturbed. Moreover, spironolactone, an end-organ receptor antagonist to aldosterone in the distal tubule, further aggravates hyperkalemia.

Diet. Diabetic patients may use salt substitutes containing potassium chloride to lower their intake of sodium chloride to treat the edema of nephrotic syndrome. During the summer, they may inc-

Table 4-2. Therapy for hyperkalemia

Agent	Regimen	Onset and duration of effect
Membrane stabilizer 10% calcium gluconate or 10%calcium chloride IV	10 mL over approximately 10 min, under cardiac monitoring	Immediate; lasts approximately 30-60 min
Shifting agents Insulin	5-10 U of regular insulin IV with 50-100 g of glucose IV (bolus), or 2-5 U/h (continuous drip) (watch patient carefully for hypoglycemia)	Within approximately 30 min; lasts a few hours
Sodium bicarbonate	1 ampule (44 mEq) IV; recheck serum pH and repeat if acidemia persists with hyperkalemia. Sodium load and hypernatremia may prohibit repeated administration. Not effective for hyperkalemia of chronic renal failure	Within minutes; lasts 1-2 h
β-Agonists	IV or nebulized albuterol; see dosage suggestions in reference 5	Within approximately 30 min; duration similar to that of insulin
Removal agents and methods Diuretics	IV furosemide (be.g.in at 40 mg and titrate for response*)	Within approximately 30-60 min; short duration; may be repeated as long as volume contraction is avoided (IV fluids may be given)
Resins	Sodium polystyrene sulfonate in sorbitol (30-60 g PO⁺); may also be given as a rectal retention enema (approximately 50 g). Do not use if ileus is present	Within hours; removes potassium during transit through GI tract (over 2-4 h)
Dialysis	Monitor if a 0 mEq/L potassium bath is used; problems less likely with a 2 mEq/L potassium bath	Immediate; removal stops as soon as dialysis stops. A 0 mEq/L potassium bath may lower the potassium level too much and precipitate hypokalemia

Presumes adequate renal function
Presumes normal GI function

rease their consumption of potassium-containing fruits and vegetables, such as tomatoes and strawberries.

Hyperglycemia. Severe hyperglycemia with or without ketoacidosis may be associated with life-threatening hyperkalemia in patients with diabetes. The mechanism is the dramatic increase in osmolality that accompanies elevated extracellular glucose concentrations. In fact, for every 10 mOsm/kg H_2O rise in the extracellular glucose concentration attributable to diabetes, the potassium concentration increases by approximately 0.6 mEq/L.

The hyperglycemia-related osmolality excess in the extracellular compartment necessitates water transfer from the intracellular compartment. Via the physical mechanism of "solvent drag," potassium passively accompanies the water as it moves to the extracellular compartment.

Since IV glucose with insulin is also used to manage hyperkalemia, iatrogenic hyperglycemia has the potential to worsen hyperkalemia. Administer 50% glucose gradually (ie, 1 ampule over 30 to 60 minutes) to avoid increasing the glucose concentration drastically.

Discussion. This patient's hyperkalemia may improve by discontinuing spironolactone and substituting a potassium-wasting diuretic (eg, furosemide). Continued treatment with the ACE inhibitor is recommended because of its benefits on renal function. Counseling about diet and the need to avoid salt substitutes may be helpful.

Remeasure the serum potassium concentration soon after changing the drug regimen to ensure that it is not rising to a potentially dangerous level. In fact, this patient's potassium level fell to 4.8 mEq/L with the described regimen, and her overall response was favorable.

Since hypoaldosteronism frequently coexists with type IV renal tubular acidosis—the only variant associated with hyperkalemia—bicarbonate may be used to lower the serum potassium level in selected outpatients. Defective renal acid secretion often accompanies the hypoaldosteronism associated with type IV renal tubular acidosis. Affected patients have a decreased serum bicarbonate level and a non-anion gap metabolic acidosis (as seen in this patient).

Excess bicarbonate (an anion) ingested orally as therapy forms complexes with sodium (a cation) in the distal nephron. As the sodium is reabsorbed, it is exchanged with potassium, which then complexes with the bicarbonate and is subsequently excreted in the urine as potassium bicarbonate. Potassium cation excretion thus increases as an obligate loss of the bicarbonate anion.

> **Table 4-3. Hyperkalemia: When it occurs in vitro but not in vivo**
>
> Spurious hyperkalemia (so-called pseudohyperkalemia) may be defined as an elevated serum potassium level that represents an in vitro but not an in vivo hyperkalemia. For example, if the platelet count is raised (eg, as in a myeloproliferative disease) when the drawn blood is allowed to clot, the intracellular potassium in the platelets (150 mEq/L) will be released into serum. (The spurious or pseudo potassium elevation detected during laboratory evaluation occurs only in drawn blood that is allowed to stand for 30 to 60 minutes before being analyzed; it does not occur in the patient.) A blood sample redrawn into a heparinized tube will usually reveal the true potassium level.
>
> Significant pseudohyperkalemia is usually discovered when platelet counts exceed 1 million/cmm. However, it may even occur to a milder degree as a consequence of venous stasis induced by prolonged use of a tourniquet.

Sodium bicarbonate taken three times daily (either as a teaspoonful dissolved in water or as tablets) may lower chronic potassium elevations while simultaneously correcting the low bicarbonate concentration associated with type IV renal tubular acidosis. Edema may be a problem because sodium bicarbonate is a salt, however. Other options (eg, Shohl's solution) are also acceptable.

CASE 4-2. Life-threatening Hyperkalemia that Masquerades as the Flu

At the outset of an influenza A epidemic, a 42-year-old man is admitted to the hospital with fever and severe muscle tenderness throughout his body. His other family members are ill with flulike symptoms; he has not been vaccinated against influenza A.

Physical examination reveals symptoms of a URI; temperature of 38.3° C (101° F); and severe, diffuse myalgias. The remainder of the examination is normal.

Electrolyte levels on admission:
      Sodium, 136 mEq/L
      Potassium, 5.6 mEq/L
      Chloride, 102 mEq/L
      Bicarbonate, 23 mEq/L
      BUN: 17 mg/dL
      Creatinine: 1.8 mg/dL

Creatinine phosphokinase: approximately twice normal with
an MM fraction elevation.

ECG: normal

Over the next 48 hours, both the muscle pain and creatinine phosphokinase MM elevation increase (the latter to approximately 20
times baseline). Urinalysis: markedly positive for blood on dipstick;
many coarsely granular casts on sediment examination; rare RBCs on
microscopic examination.

Electrolyte levels at 48 hours:
  Sodium, 132 mEq/L
  Potassium, 7.4 mEq/L
  Chloride, 96 mEq/L
  Bicarbonate, 16 mEq/L
BUN: 33 mg/dL
Creatinine: 3.8 mg/dL

Oliguria (300 mL/24 hrs) is present. Emergent ECG shows tall
peaked T waves with a prolonged QRS complex. Muscle strength is
decreased.

Discussion. The absolute potassium level and ECG changes
indicate that the patient has severe, life-threatening hyperkalemia.
Treatment must therefore be started before further workup because
of the risk of cardiac arrest.

Since the ECG shows target organ dysfunction (particularly a
prolonged QRS duration), 1 ampule (10 mL) of calcium gluconate
was administered immediately to stabilize the patient's hyperkalemic
conduction abnormality. Monitoring was required because of the
severity of the hyperkalemia. The ECG demonstrates immediate
improvement.

As mentioned, IV calcium is at best a temporizing measure and
does not remove excess potassium from the body. Consequently,
insulin (2 to 5 U/h as a continuous drip or 5 to 10 U as a bolus), 50%
glucose (50 to 100 g), and bicarbonate (1 ampule [approximately 50
mEq]) are given IV. (The bicarbonate will also correct the anion gap
metabolic acidemia that is attributable to the renal insufficiency.)

After the patient's conduction disturbance is stabilized, appropriate
diagnostic studies are performed to determine the cause of the
hyperkalemia. The influenza A infection is complicated by rhabdomyolysis (note the MM elevations accompanied by renal failure). Influenza A infection is not a common cause of rhabdomyolysis — or of
hyperkalemia, for that matter — but it is the most likely diagnosis
given this patient's elevated creatinine phosphokinase level, myalgias,

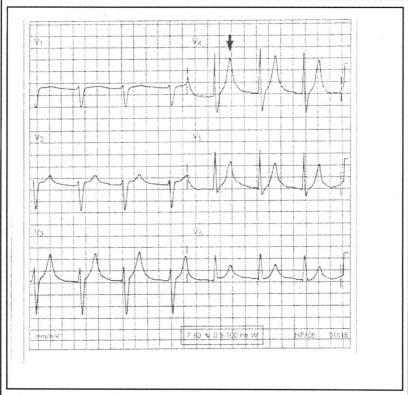

Figure 4-3. ECG of a 27-year-old patient with AIDS who is given penta-midine after Pneumocystis carinii pneumonia has been diagnosed. Note the tall peaked T waves in V^2, V^3, and V^4 (arrow) and the absence of QRS widening, indicating hyperkalemic conduction abnormalities.

renal failure, and hyperkalemia. Similar potassium elevations may develop during tumor lysis syndrome or after hemolysis (via a trans-fusion reaction or the use of "old" stored blood).

Since this patient is oliguric and is releasing large amounts of po-tassium into the circulation from injured muscle, hemodialysis against a 2 mEq/L potassium bath was required to remove the excess potas-sium. (The dialysis bath will present a potassium gradient of 5.4 mEq/L [the difference between the patient's serum potassium concen-tration of 7.4 mEq/L and the bath's potassium concentration of 2 mEq/L] for removing potassium from the body.) Over the ensuing 72 hours, myalgias and muscle injury abate, BUN and creatinine levels stabilize, and urinary output increases.

Case 4-3. Drug-induced Hyperkalemia in an AIDS Patient

A 27-year-old man with AIDS is admitted to the hospital with acute pneumonia and hypoxia. His CD4+ cell count is 150/mL. Although the patient tested positive for HIV antibody approximately a year ago, he is not currently receiving prophylaxis against *Pneumocystis carinii* pneumonia; in fact, sputum examination demonstrated *P. carinii*.

His respiration rate was 30 breaths per minute and labored. Temperature: 38.3⁰ C/(101⁰ F). Blood pressure: 90/60 mm Hg. Pulse: 110 beats per minute. Cardiac: sinus tachycardia. Chest: diffuse rales throughout both lung fields. Chest films corroborate the bilateral pneumonia.

Electrolyte levels on admission:
    Sodium, 136 mEq/L
    Potassium, 5.0 mEq/L
    Chloride, 106 mEq/L
    Bicarbonate, 19 mEq/L
BUN: normal
Creatinine: normal
Creatinine phosphokinase: approximately twice normal with an MM fraction elevation.
WBC count: 11,000/mL with a mild shift to the left (four bands)

Since the patient claims a sulfa allergy, he is given IV pentamidine (4 mg/kg/d). After 48 hours, flaccid symmetric weakness was observed in all muscle groups tested.

Electrolyte levels
    Sodium, 139 mEq/L
    Potassium, 7 mEq/L
    Chloride, 106 mEq/L
    Bicarbonate, 18 mEq/L
BUN: 21 mg/dL
Creatinine: 1.9 mg/dL
Creatinine phosphokinase: approximately twice normal with an MM fraction elevation
Urinary output: greater than 1 L/d
ECG: tall peaked T waves without widening of the QRS complexes (Figure 4-3)

Differential diagnosis. AIDS has ushered in a number of novel clinical precipitants of hyperkalemia. They include pentamidine therapy, adrenal and renal insufficiency, and hyporeninemic hypo-aldosteronism.

Pentamidine-related hyperkalemia occurs almost uniformly in AIDS patients who receive the drug for longer than 6 days. Pentamidine blocks distal tubular reabsorption of sodium, which concurrently decreases distal nephron secretion of potassium. The result: a rise in the serum potassium level that may also be accompanied by a pentamidine-induced drop in the GFR. Thus, renal potassium excretion is further compromised.

Trimethoprim-sulfamethoxazole also impairs renal potassium excretion by a mechanism similar to that of pentamidine. Consequently, one should determine serum electrolyte levels for all AIDS patients during any acute illness, especially if medications associated with hyperkalemia are used.

Discussion. Vigorous treatment — with monitoring — is indicated to stabilize this patient because of the manifest target-organ dysfunction visible on the ECG, muscle weakness, and serious elevation in the serum potassium concentration. After initial, immediate treatment with IV calcium, give IV agents to transiently shift potassium into cells and diuretics to remove excess potassium from the body. If necessary, use sodium polystyrene sulfonate or dialysis for more definitive potassium removal.

A reasonable oral dose of sodium polystyrene sulfonate is 30 g in sorbitol (conventionally mixed in the pharmacy). If bowel function is normal, dosing may be repeated approximately every 6 to 8 hours as necessary.

Before implicating pentamidine as the culprit in this patient, rule out Addison's disease and consider other possibilities in the differential. To test for Addison's disease, obtain an early-morning serum cortisol level and then give the patient 10 units of synthetic ACTH. Remeasure the serum cortisol level after 1 hour: an approximate doubling of the cortisol level suggests an adequate adrenal reserve for stress.

Suggested Reading

1. Greenberg S, Reiser IW, Chou S-Y, et al. Trimethoprim-sulfamethoxazole induces reversible hyperkalemia. *Ann Intern Med.* 1993;119:291-295.
2. Gruy-Kapral C, Emmett M, Santa Ana CA, et al. Effect of single dose resin-cathartic therapy on serum potassium concentration in patients with end-stage renal disease. *J Am Soc Nephrol.* 1998;9:1924-1930.

3.   Kleyman TR, Roberts C, Ling BN. A mechanism for pentamidine-induced hyperkalemia: inhibition of distal nephron sodium transport. *Ann Intern Med.* 1995;122:103-106.

4.   Lewis EJ, Hunsicker LG, Bain RP, et al. The effect of angiotensin-converting-enzyme inhibition on diabetic nephropathy. *N Engl J Med.* 1993;329:1456-1462.

5.   Liou HH, Chiang SS, Wu SC, et al. Hypokalemic effects of intravenous infusion of nebulization of salbutamol in patients with chronic renal failure: comparative study. *Am J Kidney Dis.* 1994;23:226-271.

6.   Potassium disorders. In: Knochel JP, ed, for the American Society of Nephrology, National Kidney Foundation, and the American College of Physicians. *MKSAP in the Subspecialty of Nephrology and Hypertension.* Philadelphia: American College of Physicians; 1994:55, 275.

7.   Rutecki GW, Whittier FC. Hypokalemia: clinical implications, consequences, and corrective measures. *Consultant.* 1996;36:124-139.

8.   Velazquez H, Perazella MA, Wright FS, Ellison DH. Renal mechanism of trimethoprim-induced hyperkalemia. *Ann Intern Med.* 1993;119:296-301.

5. Hyponatremia
Physiologic Clues to a State of Disordered Tonicity

At first glance, hypothyroidism, AIDS, and congestive heart failure may seem to have little in common. Despite the diverse pathophysiology underlying each disorder, all three may be complicated by hyponatremia. In fact, up to 25% of hospitalized patients may be hyponatremic; disordered tonicity is the most common electrolyte disturbance encountered in clinical practice. Hyponatremia also serves as a marker of disease severity in many illnesses, since hypotonicity predicts an increase in both morbidity and mortality.

In consideration of the myriad diseases associated with this disturbance, a systematic approach to the differential diagnosis of hyponatremia is essential. After the cause has been determined, keep in mind the serious complications that may occur during the attempt to correct hypotonicity. Hyponatremia that is either undertreated or overtreated may intensify the patient's condition: slight confusion may progress to symptoms of permanent CNS sequelae.

Clinical Significance

Confusion is inherent in the very term hyponatremia, for the component natremia belies the primary significance of water in both the pathophysiology of hyponatremia and any resultant CNS injury. It is not a less-than-normal value of sodium that causes problems but, rather, a greater-than-normal volume of water. Water excess leads to hypotonicity, which is a term more accurate than hyponatremia to describe the primary clinical disorder to be diagnosed and managed.

From this observation arise three corollaries. Keep these in mind as we consider the clinical variations of hyponatremia.

- First, **all true hyponatremia is dilutional,** no matter what the patient's volume status. By definition, the defect in all hyponatremic patients is too much water for body volume.

- Second, since hyponatremia is a syndrome associated with diverse and otherwise unrelated diseases, **an objective determination of volume status is essential** to simplify the clinical diagnostic workup and to define the treatment options. The relationship between volume (especially low or ineffective arterial volume) and hyponatremia is what governs stimulation of antidiuretic hormone (ADH) and resultant water retention. It is the water retention, rather than loss of sodium in excess of water in the urine, that results in clinically significant hyponatremia.

- Third, **any hyponatremia-induced CNS injury represents a change in tonicity or intracranial water content**, accompanied by swelling or shrinking in the CNS. It is not necessarily a primary change in total body water volume or sodium.

Pathophysiology

When a patient's serum sodium concentration falls below 135 mEq/L, the plasma osmolality decreases below 280 mOsm/kg water. The plasma osmolality may be determined by using an osmometer, or it may be approximated by carrying out the following calculation:

$$\frac{2[Na] + BUN + glucose}{2.6 \qquad 18} = \begin{array}{l} \text{serum} \\ \text{osmolality} \\ \text{(mOsm/kg/H}_2\text{O)} \end{array}$$

These are the three major plasma solutes that contribute to tonicity. In this formula, the serum sodium concentration is doubled because, when in solution, it is always accompanied by an anion that contributes equally to tonicity.

Pseudohyponatremia. True hyponatremia, which is an actual **decrease in plasma tonicity**, occurs whenever water in excess of solute is added to body fluids. In contrast, the term pseudohyponatremia would represent any **decrease in plasma sodium concentration** (below 135 mEq/L) without a like decrease in tonicity–ie, the plasma remains isotonic (280 mOsm/kg/H$_2$O) or is even hypertonic (greater than 280 mOsm/kg/H$_2$O). Pseudohyponatremia was not uncommon when flame photometry was used to determine sodium concentrations in the presence of hyperlipidemia, but the use of ion-specific electrodes has rendered the term almost obsolete.

Clinical example. Pseudohyponatremia (hyperosmolar hyponatremia) still can occur in patients who have diabetes mellitus. In the presence of insulin resistance or lack of insulin, each 100mg/dL increase in the serum glucose level is accompanied by a 1.6mEq/L decrease in the serum sodium level.

For example, as a diabetic patient's serum glucose concentration increases to 500 mg/dL in nonketotic hyperosmolar coma, the serum sodium level should decrease from 140 to 134 mEq/L ($1.6 \times 4 = 6.4$). This decrease represents diffusion of intracellular water into the extracellular space in response to the osmotic activity of glucose. Therefore, in the absence of hypotonicity, the condition is *pseudo*hyponatremia. In the same patient, however, a serum sodium concentration of less than 134 mEq/L would represent true hyponatremia, or water excess.

This same patient has a BUN of 20 mg/dL. Use the above-mentioned formula to calculate the osmolality:

$$\frac{2[134]}{2.6} + \frac{20}{18} + 500 = 309 \text{ mOsm/kg/H}_2\text{O}$$

Therefore, even though this patient is hyponatremic, the lowered sodium concentration would represent pseudohyponatremia because tonicity is not decreased. Other osmotically active agents associated with hypertonic hyponatremia will be discussed later.

Calculating osmolar and free water clearance. Hypotonicity in hyponatremia develops whenever water enters the body in excess of what the kidneys can excrete. Efficient excretion of water depends on adequate renal blood flow and glomerular filtration rate (GFR), adequate distal tubular diluting function, and an absence of ADH.

A simple clearance calculation will enable the understanding of this concept. The urine volume comprises osmolar clearance (cOsm) plus free water clearance. The cOsm represents the urine flow rate that is necessary to dissolve and excrete solute and waste products, such as sodium, urea, and creatinine.

If a patient drinks 2 L of water, and urine volume increases to 10 mL/min with maximum urine dilution (60 mOsm/kg/H$_2$O), the clearance formula is calculated as follows:

$$\text{cOsm} = \frac{\text{urine osmolality} \times \text{urine flow rate}}{\text{plasma osmolality}}$$

$$\text{cOsm} = \frac{60 \text{ mOsm/kg/H}_2\text{O} \times 10 \text{ mL/min}}{280 \text{ mOsm/kg/H}_2\text{O}}$$

$$= \frac{600}{280} = 2.1 \text{ mL/min}$$

The 2.1 mL/min represents the amount of water necessary to dissolve and carry out the sodium, creatinine, and BUN in the urine; free water clearance is 7.9 mL/min. In the first 4 hours, approximately 1,900 mL of free water from the 2 L ingested would be excreted in the urine.

In contrast to this instance, consider what happens when a patient who has congestive heart failure complicated by ineffective circulating arterial volume drinks 2 L of water. Volume-induced peripheral vascular constriction affects the kidneys and decreases both renal blood flow and GFR. Because of the presence of ADH, the urine osmolality will remain high at 500 mOsm/kg, and the urine flow will be only 2 mL/min. The osmolar clearance from these numbers can be calculated as follows:

$$cOsm= \frac{500 \text{ mOsm/kg/H}_2O \times 2 \text{ mL/min}}{280 \text{ mOsm/kg/H}_2O}$$

$$= \frac{1,000}{280} = 3.57$$

Urine flow rate = cOsm + free water clearance

2mL/min = 3.6 + X

Free water clearance = −1.57

Therefore, with a negative free water clearance, not only is the water load not excreted in 4 hours, but a significant amount of water is retained, leading to dilution.

Mechanisms leading to continued water reabsorption. There are three ways in which water reabsorption may be increased, thus leading to hyponatremia.

- First, any decrease in volume–real or secondary to ineffective circulating volume–increases proximal tubular reabsorption. In this situation, less filtrate reaches the distal segments of the nephron, which are responsible for dilution and water excretion.

- Second, distal nephron diluting segments must actively convey solute in excess of water to dilute the filtrate. This transport mechanism can be blunted, for example, by diuretics.

- Third, compensatory ADH release contributes to hyponatremia. ADH release occurs in response to two stimuli: hypertonicity (as expected) and volume disturbances. Hypertonicity (eg, 280 to 290 mOsm/kg/H_2O) would stimulate ADH release to increase renal water reabsorption and attenuate hypertonicity in plasma. Less recognized is the fact that decreased or ineffective arterial circulation, as perceived by the brain, also increases ADH release. Decreased volume via the release of ADH increases renal water reabsorption and dilutes plasma as a defense against further volume loss.

The continued release of ADH during CHF, for example, is often construed as being inappropriate. Yet, from a teleologic perspective, the volume response is primal; that is, the role of the kidney and of ADH is to preserve effective circulatory volume at all costs. If volume depletion or ineffective arterial circulatory volume occurs, water retention (despite development of hyponatremia) is a primary survival mechanism and, as such, it is appropriate. Dilution of plasma is the lesser of two evils, considering the outcome of continued volume depletion or ineffective circulation: hypotension and death.

Three Categories of Hyponatremia

Let us first consider the patient with hyponatremia resulting from diuretic therapy. This patient's volume status may be decreased, normal, or increased, depending on the degree of thirst and the amount of fluid ingested.

Diuretics decrease the circulating volume and thus lead to increased proximal reabsorption and decreased distal delivery of filtrate. These agents (especially thiazides) paralyze transport in distal reabsorptive sites responsible for urine dilution. Finally, diuretic-induced volume contraction stimulates ADH release, leading to further water retention. Diuretics not only cause or aggravate hyponatremia, but they confuse the urine studies used to identify the cause of hyponatremia.

Because hyponatremia may occur in multiple settings, one must develop a system to classify it. Hyponatremia is initially placed in one of three categories that are based on volume status and urinary electrolyte levels (Figure 5-1). Again, we emphasize that true hyponatremia represents excess water for an available volume, which may be low, normal, or high. The three primary categories are then subdivided according to spot urinary electrolyte determinations.

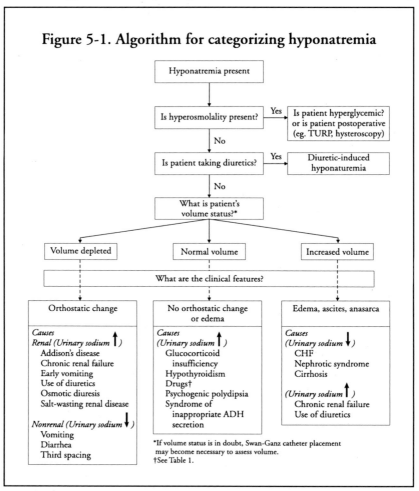

Figure 5-1. Algorithm for categorizing hyponatremia

Volume depletion. The first category, extracellular volume-depletion hyponatremia, is characterized by gastrointestinal fluid losses (from diarrhea and vomiting), diuretic-induced sodium losses, mineralo-corticoid and glucocorticoid deficiency (as in Addison's disease or primary adrenal insufficiency), or third-space losses associated with hyponatremia.

This category can be differentiated from the other two (normal volume and excess volume) by obtaining a good history and physical examination. Investigate gastrointestinal complaints, and review medication usage. Determine evidence of volume contraction from the physical examination; frequently, the only such indication is orthostatic change in blood pressure (eg, a drop of 10 mm Hg or greater in the systolic pressure, or hypotension) and pulse (increased rate).

Renal and nonrenal. Spot determinations of urinary electrolytes divide the volume depletion category of hyponatremia into renal and nonrenal subgroups. If the kidney is responsible for volume loss (eg, chronic renal failure), urinary sodium concentrations are elevated; with extrarenal loss of volume, urinary sodium concentration is low (less than 20 mEq/L). This latter situation represents avid renal retention of sodium in response to volume depletion.

Renal loss of sodium despite volume contraction suggests intrinsic renal disease, diuretic use, or Addison's disease; each of these precludes tubular sodium reabsorption in response to volume depletion. Patients with volume contraction retain water and become hyponatremic as a result of decreased renal blood flow, decreased filtrate presentation to distal sites, and stress release of ADH. Not all of them become hyponatremic, but the potential for dilution is present with water ingestion. A clinical pearl that we find useful is that the finding of a high urinary sodium excretion with hyponatremia should always prompt a search for diuretic use/abuse.

Normal volume. The second hyponatremic group is marked by excess body water in the presence of normal to modest increases in total volume. (The term "modest" is used because the volume increase does not result in edema or ascites.) Causes include endocrine disorders, such as glucocorticoid insufficiency, hypothyroidism, drugs (Table 5-1), and syndrome of inappropriate ADH secretion (SIADH). Increased ADH levels are the major cause of water retention in this group.

No postural decline in blood pressure is noted among these patients, but physical examination may uncover signs of specific diseases responsible for hyponatremia. For example, patients who have glucocorticoid deficiency due to pituitary disease may lose their axillary hair and complain of generalized weakness. Their history might reveal weight loss, anorexia, gastrointestinal symptoms, or signs of endocrine dysfunction. When hypothyroidism is the cause of hyponatremia, patients may evidence myxedematous skin changes, delayed deep tendon reflex relaxation, bradycardia, or pericardial effusion.

Table 5-1. Drugs that can cause hyponatremia

Diuretics
Antidepressants
Antipsychotics
Chemotherapeutic agents (eg, cyclophosphamide, vincristine)
Chlorpropamide
ADH-like drugs (eg, desmopressin)
Nicotine
Morphine
NSAIDs
Clofibrate
Carbamazepine

SIADH. This condition deserves a special comment: first and foremost, SIADH is a diagnosis of exclusion. Because of its similarity to hypothyroidism (hyponatremia, modest volume expansion, increase in spot urinary sodium and osmolality) make every effort to rule out other causes of hyponatremia.

Specifically, to rule out CHF, patients with SIADH should be free of edema; and their adrenal, thyroid, and renal function should be normal. Patients with SIADH show evidence of variable urinary sodium wasting (urinary sodium usually greater than 20 mEq/L) and a urine inappropriately concentrated compared with plasma hypotonicity. Urine osmolality is usually more than 300 mOsm/kg/H_2O; but with a low plasma sodium level, even 200 mOsm/kg/H_2O would be inappropriately high.

Table 5-2. Diseases associated with SIADH

Cancer
Lung (especially small-cell cancer)
Gastrointestinal (pancreas, duodenum)
Genitourinary (prostate, bladder, ureter)
Other (Ewing's sarcoma, lymphoma, mesothelioma, thymoma)

Central nervous system disorders
Infection (eg, tuberculous meningitis)
Trauma induced
Delirium tremens
Porphyria
Tumor
Hemorrhage
Stroke

Pulmonary disorders
Pneumonia
Abscess
Tuberculosis
Asthma

SIADH, syndrome of inappropriate ADH secretion

Additional laboratory studies that help differentiate SIADH from other causes of hyponatremia include measurement of serum levels of BUN, creatinine, and uric acid. The slight volume expansion in SIADH leads to heightened clearance of plasma constituents. As a result, patients who have SIADH are described as being hypouremic (low BUN and creatinine values) and hypouricemic. The concomitant presence of hypouremia and hypouricemia in a patient who has hyponatremia–particularly one lacking volume expansion or depletion–may support a diagnosis of SIADH. The diseases associated with SIADH are listed in Table 5-2.

Excess volume. In the third category of hyponatremia, patients present with volume excess, edema, ascites, and/or anasarca. This group includes the triad of CHF, nephrotic syndrome, and cirrhosis; each of which is complicated by ineffective circulating arterial volume. The triad is associated with decreased urinary sodium excretion (less than 20 mEq/L), unless diuretics have been administered or if chronic renal failure has intervened.

Conduct a physical examination focused for the particular clinical syndrome. Hyponatremia with cirrhosis may be accompanied by spider angiomas, ascites, splenomegaly, and gynecomastia. The ineffective circulating arterial volume of these three disorders leads to renal sodium retention when renal function is normal. Among these patients, water retention is caused by decreased renal blood flow, decreased GFR, and increased ADH secretion. In any of these clinical settings, ingestion of excess water will lead to hyponatremia because of the kidney's inability to excrete a water load in the presence of ADH.

If volume expansion and hyponatremia are present without a decrease in urinary sodium, consider the possibility of renal failure or diuretic use. In either circumstance, the renal injury precludes the sodium reabsorption seen in the edematous triad of patients with preserved renal function.

Hypotonic CNS Injury

The pathophysiology of brain injury in hyponatremia further substantiates the fact that hyponatremia is a water–and not a sodium–disorder. Here, any increase in water content may lead to brain expansion, resulting in serious CNS damage. Even a modest 5% increase in brain cell volume during hyponatremia may lead to herniation. The CNS compensatory mechanisms that respond to hyponatremic brain swelling are crucial to the understanding of not only hypotonicity but also its management.

As hypotonicity develops, brain cells seek to prevent excess CNS water expansion by actively decreasing intracellular osmolality. These cells can decrease their content of intracellular potassium and other solutes (perhaps by binding to protein) and thereby decrease total brain water uptake by osmotic pressure.

Nevertheless, despite this compensatory activity, hypotonic brain cells are expanded and thus are sensitive to further injury. In fact, continued water retention in untreated hyponatremia can progress from manifesting no symptoms or signs to confusion, disorientation, obtundation, coma, seizures, paralysis, and, eventually, death. Management of hypotonic brain injury with hypertonic saline can prevent progression of CNS injury. Hypertonic saline treatment, however, is the proverbial double-edged sword: its use must remain within certain parameters in order to improve CNS pathologic changes and not lead to further cell injury. These parameters will be discussed in the next chapter.

Conclusion

The diagnosis and management of hyponatremia have been clarified through a discussion of hyponatremia as a primary tonicity disturbance. The many diseases responsible for hyponatremia have been categorized according to information gathered from the patient's history and physical examination, urinary electrolyte values, and serum and urinary osmolality measurements. Clinical application was made of abnormalities in renal physiology that lead to hyponatremia. Changes in brain volume associated with hyponatremia were reviewed in preparation for a later discussion of management of hyponatremia.

Suggested Reading

1.   Ayus JC, Arieff AI. Pathogenesis and prevention of hyponatremic encephalopathy. *Endocrinol Metab Clin North Am.* 1993;22(2):425-446.

2.   Lauriat SM, Berl T. The hyponatremic patient: practical focus on therapy. *J AM Soc Nephrol.* 1997; 8:1599-1607.

3.   Steele A, Gowrishankar M, Abrahamson S, et al. Post-operative hyponatremia despite near-isotonic saline infussion: a phenomen of desalination. *Ann Intern Med.* 1997; 126: 20-25.

4.   Strange K. Regulation of solute and water balance and cell volume in the central nervous system. *J Am Soc Nephrol.* 1992;3:12-27.

5.   Vitting KE, Gardenswartz MH, Zabetakis PM, et al. Frequency of hyponatremia and nonosmolar vasopressin release in the acquired immunodeficiency syndrome. *JAMA.* 1990;263:973-978.

6. Hyponatremia
Cause of Hypotonicity
Directs Management

Despite the common thread of findings from physical examination and volume status in categorizing hyponatremia, the presence of two urinary electrolyte subgroups within the low- and high-volume groups may engender confusion. For simplification, one may utilize the three volume categories of hyponatremia with a different algorithm (Table 6-1): this incorporates the patient's volume status with physiologic interpretation of renal function, urinary electrolyte values, urine osmolality, and miscellaneous features (eg, hypouricemia, thyroid abnormalities). This approach will be illustrated by case discussions with treatment options.

CASE 6-1. Hyponatremia with Volume Contraction and Sodium Wasting

A 32-year-old man who had been ill for the past 3 months complained of loss of appetite and decreased intake, fatigue, weakness, and a 5-kg weight loss. He had had neither diarrhea nor vomiting and was not taking diuretics. His blood pressure was 90/60 mm Hg, and his pulse rate was 120 beats per minute. Intravenous fluids (normal saline) were immediately begun in the emergency department.

Laboratory studies. Serum values included sodium, 118 mEq/L; potassium 6.2 mEq/L; bicarbonate, 22 mEq/L; chloride, 86 mEq/L; BUN, 38 mg/dL; creatinine, 1.4 mg/dL, glucose, 98 mg/dL; and osmolality, 245 mOsm/kg/H_2O. Urinary values included sodium, 123 mEq/L; potassium, 15 mEq/L; and osmolality, 565 mOsm/kg/H_2O. Urinalysis results were normal.

Volume assessment. The patient's history (decreased oral intake and weight loss) and findings from his physical examination (hypotension and tachycardia) supported **severe volume contraction.** Other clues to volume contraction were laboratory data consistent with prerenal azotemia: BUN-creatinine ratio greater than 15:1. This patient's BUN-creatinine ratio of approximately 27:1, plus lack of urinary sediment, suggested poor renal perfusion as the cause of azotemia.

Kidney function. The normal renal response to volume contraction — especially to a degree severe enough to result in hypotension — is avid sodium retention and urine concentration to preclude further volume loss of sodium and water. This patient, however, had a severe degree of sodium wasting despite appropriate water reabsorption and antidiuretic hormone (ADH) effect in response to compromised circulating volume. A review of Figure 5-1, reveals the following possibilities for the paradox of volume contraction without renal salt retention:

Use of diuretics. Both thiazides and loop diuretics paralyze the nephron's ability to reabsorb sodium and potassium, interfere with concentrating and diluting ability, and may cause a contraction metabolic alkalosis. Yet this patient denied diuretic use, was hyperkalemic rather than hypokalemic, had more highly concentrated urine than plasma, and did not have a contraction metabolic alkalosis. Osmotic diuresis (eg, from glucose, urea, or mannitol) was absent, and vomiting had not occurred.

Salt-wasting nephritis and **Addison's disease** are the remaining possibilities. Salt-wasting nephritis is usually accompanied by evidence of chronic renal disease, which was not present here; the patient had a normal creatinine level and normal urinalysis. Further, he had no history of salt-wasting renal diseases, such as polycystic kidney or chronic interstitial nephritis. Addison's disease (absence of glucocorticoid and mineralocorticoid hormones due to primary adrenal failure) may lead to volume contraction, renal salt wasting, increased ADH levels, urine concentration inappropriate to plasma hypotonicity, and hyperkalemia (aldosterone is absent).

Further diagnostic workup included a corticotropin stimulation test. If the adrenal gland is functioning properly, corticotropin stimulates the adrenal output of cortisol to at least twice the baseline value. This patient had Addison's disease, and a low baseline cortisol reading was not stimulated further by corticotropin. Later, his plasma corticotropin levels were found to be elevated, which is consistent with an intact pituitary and nonfunctioning adrenal glands.

The patient's hyperkalemia, accompanied by a low urinary potassium level, represented absence of mineralocorticoid activity in the distal tubule. AIDS has been increasingly associated with adrenal insufficiency

Table 6-1. Model for diagnosis of hyponatremia

What is the patient's volume status: depleted, expanded without edema, or expanded with edema?
Is kidney function normal?
Is the kidney responding to the volume stimulus?
What is urinary osmolality? Is antidiuretic hormone present?
Is patient hypouricemic? What is thyroid status? adrenal status?

and must be considered a diagnostic possiblity here. Adrenalitis due to cytomegalovirus, mycobacterial infection, or fungal infection may be responsible for Addison's disease in a patient with AIDS. Addison's disease is one of many causes of hyponatremia in AIDS; CNS and pulmonary sources are also not uncommon.

Thus, hyponatremia with volume contraction requires consideration of physiologic parameters that include the renal response to volume contraction. Physiologic thinking leads to limited possibilities that are approached through noninvasive studies.

Therapy. This man's treatment included intravenous volume repletion with normal saline and water restriction. This also corrected the accompanying hyponatremia by rectifying the pathologic state, tonicity, and volume. Administration of normal saline was discontinued as soon as the volume deficit was corrected, but water restriction was continued.

As a rule, complications from hyponatremia correction do not occur in this group of patients. The volume of saline administered to this patient over the first 24 hours (approximately 4 L) corrected the hypotension and, combined with water restriction, increased his serum sodium level to 125 mEq/L. Also, as expected, his BUN level decreased. The replacement of corticosteroids and mineralocorticoids corrected the clinical picture, and they were continued after discharge. Water restriction was no longer required.

Case 6-2. Hyponatremia with Normal Plasma Volume and Dilute Urine

A 47-year-old woman with psychosis was readmitted because of agitation. She had discontinued her medications (lithium, haloperidol) 2 weeks earlier. Examination revealed blood pressure, 120/78 mm Hg, supine, and 130/80 mm Hg, upright; pulse, 90 beats per minute, supine, and 92 beats per minute, upright. She had no edema; results of cardiopulmonary and abdominal examinations were normal.

Laboratory studies. Serum values included sodium, 125 mEq/L; potassium, 3.8 mEq/L; bicarbonate, 25 mEq/L; chloride, 93 mEq/L; BUN, 5 mg/dL; creatinine, 0.6 mg/dL; glucose, 102 mg/dL; and osmolality, 260 mOsm/kg/H_2O. Urinary values included sodium, 8 mEq/L; potassium, 20 mEq/L; and osmolality, 60 mOsm/kg/H_2O.

Volume assessment. There was no history to support volume depletion. The examination findings were consistent with euvolemia (supine and standing blood pressure and pulse rates were normal; edema and ascites were absent).

Table 6-2. Correction of hyponatremia

Restrict water (including hypotonic IV fluids)

Discontinue medicines that may worsen hyponatremia.*

If there is end-organ CNS dysfunction from chronic hyponatremia, 3% hypertonic saline should be used with the following precautions:
- Do not allow serum sodium level to increase >0.5 mEq/h or >12 mEq/d total.
- Never attempt complete correction of serum sodium level (>125 mEq/L).
- When serum sodium level reaches ≥125 mEq/L during correction, switch from hypertonic to normal saline.

If acute hyponatremia occurs within 48 hours, (eg, postoperative syndrome in menstruant women), correct it immediately by administering hypertonic saline. (rate ~1mEq/hr)

For hyponatremia with volume contraction, administer normal saline to correct volume deficit, and restrict water.

*See Table 5-1.

Kidney function. Renal function was normal. Findings from history, physical examination, and initial laboratory work were consistent with hyponatremia and normal to slightly excess volume, without edema.

ADH status. This category is that of ADH excess. Here, urinary electrolyte levels and urinary osmolality are consistent with hyperfiltration (increased urinary sodium) and urine more highly concentrated than plasma (ADH effect). Yet, this patient's urine was at maximal dilution (60 mOsm/kg/H_2O), which suggests absence of ADH. Maximum urinary dilution and a low urinary sodium level, combined with a history of psychiatric disease and euvolemia, are associated with excess water intake, absence of ADH, and a diagnosis of psychogenic polydipsia. This is the only situation in which hyponatremia and maximal urine dilution coexist.

Therapy. Water restriction constituted adequate treatment for this patient. If CNS symptoms had been present, normal saline IV might have been given. During correction of hyponatremia, certain rules are essential to protect brain cells from osmotic injury (Table 6-2). Brain injury during hypotonicity or correction may be evaluated by a mental status examination. A change in mental status (confusion, obtundity, coma, or seizure activity) may provide evidence that hyponatremia is responsible for brain dysfunction.

Use of parenteral fluids. If patients have a CNS complication of hypotonicity, give parenteral fluids in addition to restricting oral water intake. You will need to know what solution to use, how to calculate the amount to be given, and how fast to correct the tonicity disturbance (in light of alterations in brain osmolality regulation). First, always restrict water, oral and parenteral, when CNS disturbance is evident on physical examination.

Solution strength. Use normal saline when possible. Reserve hypertonic saline (3%) for more serious CNS disturbance (confusion, obtundation, seizures, or acute changes in tonicity occurring in less than 48 hours).

Amount given. The excess water in hyponatremia occupies both extracellular and intracellular compartments. Thus, calculate correction for total body water space and not for extracellular space alone.

Degree and rate of correction. Never correct the hyponatremic disturbance completely, and never correct chronic hyponatremia to more than 125 mEq/L or by more than 12 mEq in 24 hours. More complete correction of hypotonicity may be complicated by development of permanent neurologic sequelae.[2,3]

To protect against further brain injury during correction of hypotonicity, administer hypertonic or normal saline IV cautiously. Do not exceed a 0.5mEq/h increase in the serum sodium concentration (or a total of 12 mEq/d). As soon as possible, discontinue IV saline and restrict water orally.

CASE 6-3. Hyponatremia with Euvolemia

A 62-year-old man, who smoked one pack of cigarettes daily for 40 years, was admitted to the hospital in a state of confusion that progressed to obtundation. Four months earlier, small-cell cancer of the lung had been diagnosed.

The patient weighed 70 kg. His blood pressure was 140/90 mm Hg, and his pulse was 96 beats per minute. He was afebrile, but he was too ill to stand up and could be aroused only by pain. Meningismus, jugular venous distension, and focal neurologic abnormalities were absent.

Heart examination revealed an audible S_4; the patient's lungs were clear to percussion and auscultation. No abnormalities were noted on the abdominal and peripheral examination, and the patient had no edema. He had been taking no medications before being admitted. Findings from a CT scan of the brain and a lumbar puncture were normal.

Laboratory studies. Serum values included sodium, 108 mEq/L; potassium, 3.2 mEq/L; bicarbonate, 23 mEq/L; chloride, 76 mEq/L; BUN, 3 mg/dL; creatinine, 0.4 mg/dL; uric acid, 2 mg/dL; glucose, 90 mg/dL; osmolality, 226 mOsm/kg/H_2O. Urinary electrolytes included sodium, 66 mEq/L; potassium, 20 mEq/L; and osmolality, 560 mOsm/kg/H_2O.

Three weeks earlier, the patient's serum sodium level had been 132 mEq/L. Additional laboratory values included a normal serum concentration of thyroid-stimulating hormone, a normal cortisol response (increased by a factor of 3) to corticotropin stimulation, and a normal urinalysis.

Volume assessment. The patient demonstrated neither volume excess (no abnormalities on heart examination, no jugular venous distention, lungs clear, and no peripheral edema) nor volume depletion (slight hypertension rather than hypotension). His history suggests adequate oral intake. The patient was euvolemic without edema.

Causes of hyponatremia in this category include drugs, hypothyroidism, glucocorticoid insufficiency, psychogenic polydipsia, and the syndrome of inappropriate ADH secretion (SIADH). The patient's workup and laboratory data exclude all but the last disorder, leading to a diagnosis of SIADH. Further, the hyponatremia is accompanied by urinary osmolality higher than that of serum, an elevated urinary sodium level, and both hypouremia and hypouricemia. The diagnosis of SIADH is also consistent with small-cell carcinoma of the lung.

Therapy. The pertinent question now was, how should this patient be treated: with isotonic or hypertonic saline or with water restriction alone? There was evidence of end-organ dysfunction (obtundation), and it had developed over a relatively short time period; therefore, he required parenteral (but cautious) treatment.[4,5]

Hypertonic saline was chosen, with the intent of correcting the hyponatremia by 6 mEq in the first 12 hours (increasing the sodium level from 108 to 114 mEq/L) or by 12 mEq in the first 24 hours (to a level of 120 mEq/L), calculated as follows:

- A 12 mEq increase in sodium concentration (from 108 to 120 mEq/L) in the first 24 hours would occur in a 70 kg adult, who has approximately 42 L of total body water (60% of body weight).
- An increase of 12 mEq in a 42 L space is approximately 500 mEq of osmotic activity (42×12).
- Since normal saline is 0.9% NaCl, 1 L of normal saline contains 154 mEq of sodium; 1 L of 3% saline thus contains approximately 500 mEq of sodium ($3 \times 154 = 462$; $462 \div 0.9 = 513.3$).

- This particular patient would thus require approximately 30 mL of 3% saline per hour to achieve a 12 mEq/L correction in the first 24 hours. At 30 mL/h, the total amount of sodium falls short of the predicted correction volume, but this figure was chosen for safety. If you are in doubt, always correct chronic hyponatremia conservatively, but do not hesitate to use hypertonic saline when there is significant CNS dysfunction.

During administration of hypertonic saline, check serum electrolyte levels every 2 hours. Adjustments in the administration rate are mandatory when indicated, as are frequent mental status examinations. After correction has been achieved (remember: only *approximate* 125 mEq/L), continue water restriction and discontinue parenteral treatment.

Following his discharge, this patient's treatment might include continued water restriction and administration of declomycin; this tetracycline antibiotic is associated with a nephrogenic diabetes insipidus syndrome (antagonism to excess ADH effect). It may, therefore, block the inappropriate urine concentration that led to hyponatremia. Do not prescribe thiazide diuretics for such a patient, as they would interfere with distal tubular diluting function and further compromise water excretion.

Avoiding Dangers of Iatrogenic Hyponatremia

Severe, rapid, life-threatening hyponatremia may develop in four types of patients:

- Elderly persons who are taking diuretics
- Menstruant women receiving hypotonic IV fluids during and following surgery
- Any postoperative hospitalized patient who is in pain, has elevated ADH levels, and is receiving dilute fluids and incriminating medications
- Patients undergoing hysteroscopy or TURP who are receiving a hypotonic glycine irrigation

The first two groups of patients mentioned are particularly prone to permanent neurologic injury and death from hypotonicity.

The second group (young women, following surgery) especially may benefit from rapid correction of hyponatremia, since hypotonicity may develop within a short period. Prompt correction prevents the brain solute loss seen with chronic hyponatremia and lessens complications with hypertonic saline correction. Nevertheless, all four groups of patients would be best protected by avoidance of thiazides and hypotonic fluids in situations associated with elevated ADH levels and water retention.

CASE 6-4. Acute Postoperative Hyponatremia

A 72-year-old man was a routine admission for transurethral resection of the prostate (TURP). A six-month history of urinary frequency, hesitancy and decreased stream led to terazosin treatment initially with some improvement. However, a persistent urinary residual of over 200 cc and a recent urinary tract infection led to admission. The prostate specific antigen (PSA) was normal. His surgery was uncomplicated, but he became confused and restless 4 hours postoperatively.

Exam. Blood pressure 140/94; pulse 98; temperature 98.6°F, respirations 20. He is disoriented, but without focal neurologic findings. Cardiac, pulmonary and abdominal exams are unremarkable.

Laboratory data. Sodium, 108 mEq/dL; potassium, 3.4 mEq/dL; chloride, 70 mEq/dL; bicarbonate, 20 mEq/dL; BUN, 12 mg/dL; Creatinine, 1.1 mg/dL. Serum osmolality, 310 mOsm/kg/H_2O. A preoperative sodium was 142 mEq/dL.

Although not common, acute post-operative hyponatremia may complicate two settings: after hysteroscopic surgery in females and after TURP in males. The culprit is the glycine and water used to irrigate the operative bed. One prospective study in one hundred TURP patients demonstrated hyponatremia in seven; one patient died as a result. In females with post-hysteroscopic hyponatremia in the setting of endometrial ablation, hyponatremia is also seen with significant morbidity and mortality.

Absorption of the glycine solution used for irrigation expands extracellular volume so that some of the glycine enters cells and is then metabolized. Unfortunately, glycine metabolic products include serine, ammonia and oxalic acid — all of which are toxic.

Treatment is controversial since some patients sustain central nervous system dysfunction from hypotonic hyponatremia while others have isotonic or even hypertonic hyponatremia (our patient). Hypertonic saline is reasonable in the setting of severe hypotonicity (as it is for other hypotonic-hyponatremias with CNS dysfunction), but seems inappropriate for hypertonic hyponatremia with an osmolar gap (from circulating, absorbed glycine). Dialysis may be a reasonable alternative in this instance to remove glycine and correct the hyponatremia.

Conclusion

Presentation of these four patients facilitates the diagnosis and management of hyponatremia from multiple causes. Information from the history and physical examination is used to determine volume status, urinary electrolyte levels, and concentration data further categorizing the abnormality. Treatment with water restriction, normal saline, and hypertonic saline is reviewed in the context of CNS toxicity. Cautious parameters are outlined in use of hypertonic saline to prevent worsening of the CNS injury seen in hyponatremia. Rapid correction of hyponatremia is discussed for groups of patients prone to acute water retention.

Suggested Reading

1. Agarwal R, Emmett M. The post-transurethral resection of prostate syndrome: therapeutic proposals. *Am J Kid Dis.* 1994;24:108-111.
2. Ayus JC, Wheeler JM, Arieff AI. Postoperative hyponatremic encephalopathy in menstruant women. *Ann Intern Med.* 1992;117:891-897.
3. Fraser CL, Arieff AI. Epidemiology, pathophysiology and management of hyponatremic encephalopathy. *Am J Med.* 1997;102:67-77.
4. Laureno R, Karp BI. Myelinolysis after correction of hyponatremia. *Ann Intern Med.* 1997;126:57-62.
5. Sterns RH, Cappuccio JD, Silver SM, Cohen EP. Neurologic sequelae after treatment of severe hyponatremia: a multicenter perspective. *J Am Soc Nephrol.* 1994;4(8):1522-1530.
6. Zarinetchi F, Berl T. Evaluation and management of severe hyponatremia. *Adv Intern Med.* 1996;41:241-283.

7. Hypernatremia
Misunderstood and Dangerous

In the day-to-day practice of medicine, it is common to see electrolyte disorders such as a low serum sodium level, high or low potassium levels, acid-base derangements, and abnormalities of calcium and magnesium. An elevated serum sodium concentration, on the other hand, appears only now and then and is, therefore, the most poorly understood electrolyte disorder of the adult. Hypernatremia deserves thorough study, because its clinical syndrome may be severe.

Clinical Presentation

The two principal causes of hypernatremia are net water loss without electrolyte loss and net sodium retention without water retention. In almost all cases, the loss of water or the excessive sodium retention is relative rather than an absolute increase in either: excessive water loss merely exceeds sodium loss, or excessive sodium intake outstrips water intake.

Etiology

The most common prelude to hypernatremia is altered consciousness — usually stupor or coma — during which a patient stops drinking water altogether. Some comatose patients also are vomiting, are febrile, are diaphoretic, or are on mechanical ventilation, adding further to water loss and relative sodium excess. Deliberate dehydration to reduce the risk of intracranial herniation and steroid-induced Cushing's syndrome encourage the development of hypernatremia.

A serum sodium concentration almost never exceeds 155 mEq/L in an alert patient with an intact thirst mechanism and adequate water supply. Even with diabetes insipidus, thirst plays the predominant role to prevent hypernatremia, and a patient often drinks 15 to 20 liters of fluids a day to match urine output. Exceptional instances in which altered consciousness does not precede water loss are essential hypernatremia and excessive adrenal corticoid activity.

Hypernatremia rarely results from a single cause. Most cases reflect the combined effects of several of the conditions mentioned above. The etiology of hypernatremia divides to cover conditions that lead directly to water loss and those that lead to sodium retention. The single exception to this classification scheme is idiopathic essential hypernatremia.

Symptoms

Many clinicians believe hypernatremia becomes symptomatic only if the serum sodium level rises abruptly over 160 mEq/L or gradually over 170 mEq/L. The symptoms are primarily neurologic: lethargy and confusion, twitching, grand mal seizures, stupor, and coma. Obviously, one of the diagnostic challenges is to determine whether a patient's altered consciousness was a cause of hypernatremia, a result of hypernatremia, or both.

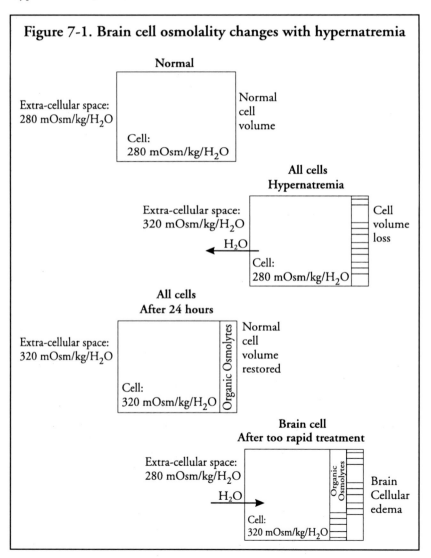

Figure 7-1. Brain cell osmolality changes with hypernatremia

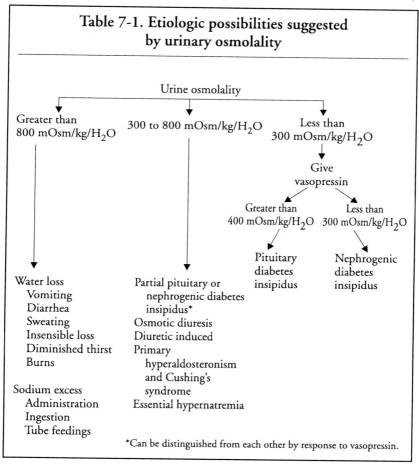

Table 7-1. Etiologic possibilities suggested by urinary osmolality

Urine osmolality		
Greater than 800 mOsm/kg/H_2O	300 to 800 mOsm/kg/H_2O	Less than 300 mOsm/kg/H_2O
		Give vasopressin
		Greater than 400 mOsm/kg/H_2O → Pituitary diabetes insipidus / Less than 300 mOsm/kg/H_2O → Nephrogenic diabetes insipidus

Water loss
  Vomiting
  Diarrhea
  Sweating
  Insensible loss
  Diminished thirst
  Burns
 	
Sodium excess
  Administration
  Ingestion
  Tube feedings
	Partial pituitary or
	  nephrogenic diabetes
	  insipidus*
	Osmotic diuresis
	Diuretic induced
	Primary
	  hyperaldosteronism
	  and Cushing's
	  syndrome
	Essential hypernatremia	

*Can be distinguished from each other by response to vasopressin.

If you suspect hypernatremia, measure the serum sodium level; a level greater than 150 mEq/L usually is not difficult to establish. You'll also want to document urinary osmolality, which can help to uncover the underlying cause of hypernatremia (Table 7-1).

Major symptoms of hypernatremia are attributed to increased extracellular osmolality. This condition draws out water from cells in the brain, resulting in dehydration of brain tissues (Figure 7-1). Associated necrosis and rupture of small vessels within the brain may lead to permanent focal neurologic deficits.

With acute hypernatremia, brain cells react quickly — within 24hrs — to produce osmotically active intracellular ions (organic osmolytes), which increase intracellular osmolality and return brain-cell fluid volume to normal. Production of these osmolytes is a mystery that seems to be

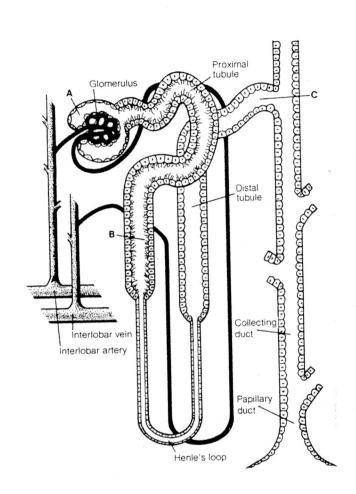

Figure 7-2. The three major physiologic functions that influence sodium reabsorption within a renal tubule are diminished glomerular filtration (A), inhibition of natriuresis along the proximal tubule (B), and aldosterone-induced sodium reabsorption along the distal tubule (C).

unique to the brain. Cells of the rest of the body remain dehydrated in hyperosmolar states, which may partially explain the profound muscle weakness with hypernatremia.

Specific Hypernatremic Syndromes

Nephrogenic or Pituitary Diabetes Insipidus

Hypernatremia may occur secondary to diabetes insipidus because antidiuretic hormone (ADH) either is not produced by the hypothalamic portion of the brain (pituitary) or is ineffective at the kidney (nephrogenic). The result in both cases is continuous diuresis of up to 25 to 30 liters per day and stimulation of all three sodium resorption mechanisms (Figure 7-1).

Patients with diabetes insipidus rarely become hypernatremic, though, owing to an intact thirst mechanism. Again, altered consciousness or some intracranial pathology must precede water loss. Occasionally the precipitating factor is administration of salt-containing I.V. fluids.

Pituitary diabetes insipidus can be easily distinguished from the nephrogenic form, and from other causes of hypernatremia, by measuring urine osmolality. If urine osmolality is less than 300 mOsm/kg/H_2O, administer 5 units of aqueous vasopressin (ADH) subcutaneously; if urine osmolality then increases to 400 mOsm/kg/H_2O or more, suspect pituitary diabetes insipidus. A patient with nephrogenic diabetes insipidus will exhibit no increase in urine osmolality due to vasopressin challenge.

Even if urine osmolality is between 300 and 800 mOsm/kg/H_2O, consider administration of vasopressin to help distinguish between partial pituitary or nephrogenic diabetes. Some medications can cause effects that mimic diabetes insipidus and sometimes they are associated with hypernatremia; such drugs include lithium, demeclocycline, propoxyphene, methoxyflurane, furosemide, and ethacrynic acid.

Osmotic or diuretic hypernatremia

Excessive osmotic diuresis can cause hypernatremia. Urea often works its osmotic effect in patients with recently relieved urinary tract obstruction; up to 1 liter of dilute urine per hour may result. An identical diuresis problem sometimes occurs post-operatively in renal transplant recipients.

An elevated plasma glucose level also can cause hypernatremia through osmotic diuresis and sodium retention. Measurement of the serum sodium rarely yields a value above the normal, however, because the value is masked. A clinical rule of thumb is that for each 100 mg/dl elevation of glucose above the normal 100 mg/dL, the measured serum

---

Table 7-2. Calculation of water deficit

Step 1. Figure that total body water content is 60% of total body weight.

$$60 \text{ kg} \times 60\% = 36 \text{ liters}$$
$$70 \text{ kg} \times 60\% = 42 \text{ liters}$$
$$80 \text{ kg} \times 60\% = 48 \text{ liters}$$

Step 2. Because extracellular and intracellular osmolality are equal under normal conditions; you can calculate the normal total cation concentration (sodium and potassium) by multipyling the normal serum sodium concentration by the normal body water content.

$$36 \text{ liters} \times 140 \text{ mEq/L} = 5040$$
$$42 \text{ liters} \times 140 \text{ mEq/L} = 5880$$
$$48 \text{ liters} \times 140 \text{ mEq/L} = 6720$$

Step 3. Divide the measured serum sodium concentration into the total cation number obtain the volume of actual body water content.

$$5040 \div 160 \text{ mEq/L} = 31.5 \quad \text{liters}$$
$$5880 \div 160 \text{ mEq/L} = 36.75 \quad \text{liters}$$
$$6720 \div 160 \text{ mEq/L} = 42 \quad \text{liters}$$

Step 4. Simply subtract the actual body water content from the normal body water content to figure the deficit. Even large variations in the inital estimate of acutal body water volume or weight have little effect on the final water deficit calculation.

$$36 - 31.5 = 4.5 \quad \text{liter water deficit}$$
$$42 - 36.75 = 5.25 \text{ liter water deficit}$$
$$48 - 42 = 6.0 \quad \text{liter water deficit}$$

---

sodium values reduce by 1.5 to 3 mEq/L (usual 1.6) as a result of water transfer out of cells.

You can calculate the degree of masked hypernatremia by multiplying 1.6 mEq/liter by the number of 100 mg/dL increments of glucose above the normal 100 mg/dL and adding the resultant to the measured serum sodium value. For example, if a diabetic patient presents with a serum glucose value of 1100 mg/dL and a serum sodium of 126 mEq/L, multiply 1.6 times 10 and add to 126 to give a value of 156 mEq/L.

We have seen serum sodium concentrations as high as 175 mEq/L. Understandably, patients with hyperosmolar or ketotic coma and high calculated sodium concentrations should be treated with hypotonic fluids and not normal saline (154 mEq/L). If insulin alone were used for treatment and normal saline were given for fluid replacement, profound hypernatremia could result.

Factors that occasionally cause hypernatremia include excessive urea removal with hyperosmolar (high-glucose-containing) peritoneal dialysis fluid. Exogenous osmotic agents, such as mannitol, given continuously or in excessive amounts, have also been reported to cause hypernatremia.

Excessive Sodium Retention

Conditions that cause hypernatremia in adults through excessive sodium retention are rare. Some patients, though, given large amounts of sodium bicarbonate during cardiac resuscitation may experience transient hypernatremia. If renal hypoperfusion and cardiac failure develop, the hypernatremia may persist and, occasionally, dialysis is the only appropriate treatment. We also recommend that you avoid the use of hypertonic sodium chloride (3% or 5%), except for rare instances of severe hyponatremia with mental status changes. Otherwise there is danger of too fast a correction of the serum sodium.

Some patients who exercise in hot climates experience hypernatremia if they ingest salt tablets without adequate water intake.

Theoretically, primary hyperaldosteronism and Cushing's syndrome can cause hypernatremia because the excess of mineralocorticoid in both syndromes causes continuous distal tubular sodium resorption and concomitant loss of potassium and hydrogen ions. However, to our knowledge, there has never been a report of a patient with either primary hyperaldosteronism or Cushing's syndrome presenting with a serum sodium above 160 mEq/L.

A patient occasionally presents with idiopathic hypernatremia, generally with serum sodium measurement in the range of 152 to 160 mEq/L but sometimes as high as 180 mEq/L. Some clinicians suggest that the cause is an inability of the CNS osmole receptor to recognize a change in serum osmolality, leaving only CNS volume receptors to regulate serum volume and concentration. This amounts to partial pituitary diabetes insipidus.

Others argue that this syndrome is a result of a "reset osmostat": a patient concentrates and dilutes urine in response to a new, higher osmolar range but within the limits of the narrow normal body response to osmolality of 1 to 2 mOsm/kg/H_2O. There may actually be two different types of patients. In either event, these patients appear normal and do not require treatment.

Treatment Decisions

If water loss is the primary clinical problem (and it usually is), replace fluids orally, or, if a patient is unconscious, by intravenous administration

---

Table 7-3. Maximum fluid replacement in a 6-hour period

If a patient has a serum sodium concentration of 170 mEq/L and a body weight of 70 kg, calculate actual body water content:

$$70 \times 60\% = 42 \text{ liters (normal body water)}$$
$$42 \times 140 \text{ mEq/L} = 5880 \text{ (normal cation content)}$$
$$5880 \div 170 \text{ mEq/L} = 34.6 \text{ liters (actual body water)}$$

To avoid an extreme osmolar gradient across brain cell membranes, correct the serum sodium concentration to 160 mEq/L over the first 6hrs (a net change of only 10 mEq/L). To calculate the amount of water needed to correct the serum sodium concentration, substitute 160 for 170 in the equation; the new "actual body water" is 36.75 liters.

$$36.75 - 34.6 = 2.15 \text{ liters (the amount of water needed to reduce sodium concentration to 160)}$$

Make similar calculations over the following 6-hour periods until a normal serum sodium concentration is reached.

---

of 5% dextrose and water. Rather than giving water empirically, calculate the water deficit. If accurate data are available, the easiest way to calculate water deficit is to determine weight loss.

Another method of estimating water deficit is to judge the severity of symptoms. Obtundation and imminent cardiovascular collapse usually signal a 10% loss of body fluid. Because of patient variability, however, and the possibility that symptoms are associated with the underlying disease and not the hypernatremia, errors may result by this estimation.

Assuming hypernatremia is related only to water loss with the total body cation content unchanged, the best method of calculating water loss is a mathematical formula based on the measured serum sodium concentration and an estimate of the normal body fluid space for a particular patient (Table 7-2).

Once one has determined the water deficit, a favorable rate of fluid administration should be chosen according to the severity of symptoms. As a rule, administer fluids gradually over 48hrs or longer to avoid overloading plasma volume and to avoid causing cerebral edema by rapid correction of the extracellular osmolality.

Clinically significant transmembrane water shifts require an osmolar gradient of 30 mOsm (15 mEq/L change in serum sodium). Therefore, avoid altering the serum sodium concentration by more than 15 mEq/L in 6hrs. Calculate maximum fluid replacement in a 6-hour period with the same methodology used to find water deficit (Table 7-3). Allow for an additional amount of water — usually 30 to 40 mL/hr — to compensate for insensible and urinary losses of body fluids.

After initiating fluid replacement, turn your efforts toward correcting the underlying cause of the hypernatremia. With pituitary diabetes insipidus, administer vasopressin to stop water loss. With hyperosmolar or ketotic diabetic coma, try to control blood sugar to reduce plasma osmolality and prevent osmolar diuresis.

CASE 7-1. Ingestion of Salt Tablets without Adequate Water Intake

One summer, a novice tennis player was brought to the emergency room after he exercised for 2hrs at 107°F (he had been told that this would improve his stamina). He had taken salt tablets, lost about 7 kg of body weight through sweating, and had not replenish his fluid losses. He was confused and his serum sodium was 171 mEq/L. He had a body temperature of 99°F, profound muscle weakness, and myoclonus. The patient responded well to rapid hydration with oral hypotonic fluids (water and Seven-Up).

CASE 7-2. Pneumonia with Altered State of Consciousness

A 77-year-old resident of a nursing home is admitted to the hospital with a three-day history of change in mental status. The patient was unable to give a history or review of systems. On physical examination the vital signs revealed a blood pressure of 100/60, pulse, 110; respirations, 14/min, and a temperature of 101°F. The neck was supple. Rales and dullness to percussion were noted at the right base posteriorly. The heart was significant for sinus tachycardia without murmurs, rubs or abnormal sound. There was slight tenting of the skin and no ankle edema. Laboratory studies included:

> Sodium, 168 mEq/L
> Potassium, 4.6 mEq/L
> Chloride, 120 mEq/L
> Bicarbonate, 30 mEq/L
> Glucose, 104 mg/dL
> BUN, 34 mg/dL
> Creatinine, 2.2 mg/dL

The CBC was within normal limits. Chest X-Ray was compatible with right lower lobe pneumonia.

The diagnosis of hypernatremia and pneumonia were established. Causes for the increased sodium level include fever with the bacterial infection (insensible loss of water) and lack of access to water with the altered state of consciousness.

In correcting the hypernatremia of the elderly, too rapidly (one day or less) is associated with a higher mortality than too slowly (greater than four days). This patient was gradually corrected over a three-day period utilizing the formulas in Table 7-2 to replace the water deficiency. Antibiotics were added to treat the pneumonia, and the patient had a complete recovery to her baseline mental status.

Hyperatremia is most commonly seen in this type of geriatric patient presentation and accounts for the greater majority of all instances of hypernatremia.

Summary

Hypernatremia is a rare but dangerous electrolyte disorder. An accurate diagnosis of the underlying cause aids therapy. By paying careful attention both to the amount of body fluid lost and to the appropriate rate of fluid replacement, one can readily correct the problem in most instances.

Suggested Reading

1.   Borra SI, Beredo R, Kleinfeld M. Hypernatremia in the aging: causes, manifestations, and outcome. *J Nat Med Assoc.* 1995; 87:220-224.

2.   Kumar S, Berl T. Sodium. *Lancet.* 1998; 352(9123):220-228.

3.   McManus ML, Churchwell KB, Strange K. Regulation of cell volume in health and disease. N Engl J Med. 1995; 1260-1265.

4.   Palevsky PM. Hypernatremia. *Semin Nephrol.* 1998; 18(1):20-30.

5.   Singer I, Oster JR, Fishgman LM. The management of diabetes insipidus in adults. Arch Intern Med. 1997; 157:1293-1302.

6.   Vieweg V, Lombana A, Lewis R. Hyper- and hyponatremia among geropsychiatric inpatients. *J Geriatr Psychiatry Neurol* 1994; 7(3):148-152.

8. Hypocalcemia
Is Emergent Therapy Required?

Hypocalcemia can be both the cause and the consequence of critical illness. Low serum calcium levels can lead to neuromuscular abnormalities (such as muscle weakness, tetany, and seizures); respiratory problems (such as bronchospasm, laryngospasm, and respiratory failure); and cardiac-related complications (such as hypotension, ventricular arrhythmias, and cardiac arrest). Hypocalcemia also can result from diverse disorders, such as sepsis, pancreatitis, toxic shock syndrome, and rhadbomyolysis. Furthermore, in critically ill patients, a serum calcium level below 8 mg/dL is often considered a marker of disease severity.

Thus, the early recognition and treatment of hypocalcemia can be an essential component of the management of critical illness. However, because 40% of serum calcium is protein-bound, standard laboratory measures of total serum calcium may not accurately reflect true hypocalcemia — that is, low levels of the ionized fraction. In addition, signs and symptoms of hypocalcemia may not always be present.

CASE 8-1. A 35-year-old Man with Chronic Alcoholism

A 35-year-old man with a long history of alcohol abuse was admitted to the hospital for severe abdominal pain accompanied by nausea and vomiting. Rebound tenderness and signs of peritonitis were absent. The abdominal pain increased when the patient was in the supine position. Bowel sounds were decreased; no rectal abnormalities were noted. Other physical findings included blood pressure, 98/60 mm Hg; pulse, 110 beats per minute and regular; respiratory rate, 20 breaths per minute and slightly labored; and temperature, normal.

Initial laboratory tests revealed the following values: sodium, 146 mEq/L; potassium, 2.9 mEq/L; chloride, 111 mEq/L; calcium, 8.8 mg/dL; phosphorus, 2.4 mg/dL; albumin, 3.9 g/dL; magnesium, 1 mEq/L; glucose, 210 mg/dL; bicarbonate, 19 mEq/L; blood urea nitrogen (BUN), 35 mg/dL; creatinine, 1.2 mg/dL; amylase, 400 U/L; lipase, 205 U/L; lactate dehydrogenase, 450 U/L; aspartate aminotransferase, 80 U/L; and alanine aminotransferase, 56 U/L.

In addition, the patient's white blood cell count was 17,000/mL, with 98% polymorphonuclear leukocytes; the hemoglobin level was 17 g/dL. Blood gas analysis showed: arterial pH, 7.32; arterial oxygen tension, 78 mm Hg; and arterial carbon dioxide tension, 30 mm Hg.

A chest film showed a small right pleural effusion. The ECG was normal. Ultrasonographic findings of the abdomen included ileus and was consistent with acute pancreatitis, without gallstones or biliary tract obstruction.

Within 48 hours of admission, the patient's abdominal pain increased, bowel sounds disappeared, and his body temperature rose to 38.3°C (101°F). In addition, the patient complained of circumoral numbness. Both Chvostek's sign and Trousseau's sign were positive.

Laboratory tests revealed a total serum calcium level of 7 mg/dL; the level of ionized calcium was low, 1.84 mEq/L. Other findings included phosphorus, 3 mg/dL; magnesium, 0.9 mEq/L; and albumin 2.9 g/dL. An ECG showed a prolonged QT interval.

Is the hypocalcemia real? The first concern is whether the low serum calcium level reflects true hypocalcemia (algorithm). The serum albumin level decreased by 1 mg/dL over the first 48 hours; thus, the total serum calcium level should have dropped by 0.8 mg/dL, to 8 mg/dL. (For an explanation of how to adjust the total serum calcium level for changes in serum protein concentration, see Chapter 9, "Hypercalcemia: The '3-hormone, 3-organ rule.'") Instead, it dropped to 7 mg/dL. At 1.84 mEq/L, the serum level of ionized calcium also was low; normal values range from 2.26 to 2.64 mEq/L. Therefore, both calcium values are consistent with true hypocalcemia.

Gentle tapping over the patient's facial nerve elicited muscle irritability, marked by fasciculations (Chvostek's sign). Also, a carpal spasm developed following compression of his forearm by a blood pressure cuff that occluded circulation for approximately 1 minute (Trousseau's sign). Both these signs indicate neuromuscular irritability and, in the present patient, support the diagnosis of true hypocalcemia.

Is end-organ dysfunction present? Usually, the next step in evaluating hypocalcemia is to measure the parathyroid hormone (PTH) level. However, when complications of hypocalcemia (such as tetany, neuromuscular irritability, hypotension, seizures, and ECG abnormalities) are evident, emergent treatment is required.

Elemental calcium (10 to 30 mL of 10% calcium gluconate) diluted in 150 mL of 5% dextrose in water can be given intravenously over approximately 10 minutes. More rapid infusions may lead to bradycardia and asystole. The therapeutic effect lasts for approximately 2 hours.

If the patient's hypocalcemia persists, a continuous infusion of calcium may be required. The recommended infusion rate for calcium gluconate ranges from 0.3 to 2 mg/kg/h. It should be emphasized,

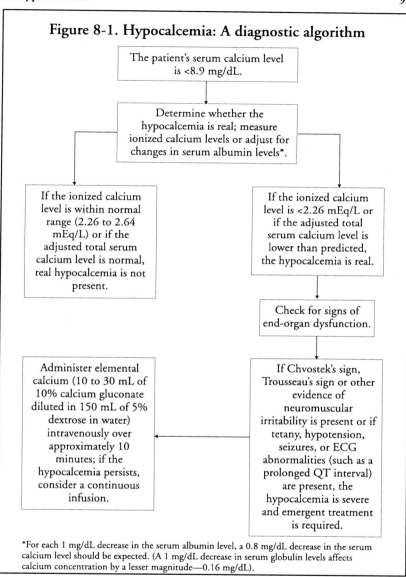

Figure 8-1. Hypocalcemia: A diagnostic algorithm

The patient's serum calcium level is <8.9 mg/dL.

Determine whether the hypocalcemia is real; measure ionized calcium levels or adjust for changes in serum albumin levels*.

If the ionized calcium level is within normal range (2.26 to 2.64 mEq/L) or if the adjusted total serum calcium level is normal, real hypocalcemia is not present.

If the ionized calcium level is <2.26 mEq/L or if the adjusted total serum calcium level is lower than predicted, the hypocalcemia is real.

Check for signs of end-organ dysfunction.

Administer elemental calcium (10 to 30 mL of 10% calcium gluconate diluted in 150 mL of 5% dextrose in water) intravenously over approximately 10 minutes; if the hypocalcemia persists, consider a continuous infusion.

If Chvostek's sign, Trousseau's sign or other evidence of neuromuscular irritability is present or if tetany, hypotension, seizures, or ECG abnormalities (such as a prolonged QT interval) are present, the hypocalcemia is severe and emergent treatment is required.

*For each 1 mg/dL decrease in the serum albumin level, a 0.8 mg/dL decrease in the serum calcium level should be expected. (A 1 mg/dL decrease in serum globulin levels affects calcium concentration by a lesser magnitude—0.16 mg/dL).

however, that calcium gluconate differs from calcium chloride in two important respects. Calcium gluconate is less irritating to blood vessels than calcium chloride. Also, compared with calcium gluconate, each gram of calcium chloride contains approximately three times more elemental calcium.

What does hypocalcemia signify in this patient? Hypocalcemia in a patient who has acute pancreatitis is a negative prognostic sign. A serum calcium concentration of less than 8 mg/dL at 48 hours after admission is one of Ranson's criteria for disease severity (Table 8-1). Recently, the APACHE II score also has been used to grade the severity of pancreatitis.

A number of theories (none proven but all plausible) have been proposed to explain the relationship between pancreatitis and hypocalcemia, including:

- Saponification of calcium (the bonding of calcium to necrotic fats)
- An increase in calcitonin levels resulting from pancreatic glucagon release (calcitonin lowers serum calcium levels by decreasing osteoclast activity and stimulating calciuresis)

Table 8-1. Ranson's criteria for pancreatitis severity

On admission:
Age >55 years
WBC count > 16,000 mL
Serum glucose level >200 mg/dL
Serum LDH level >350 U/L
Serum AST level >250 U/L

After 48 hours:
Hematocrit decrease of >10%
BUN increase of >5 mg/dL
Serum calcium level <8 mg/dL
PaO_2 <60 mm Hg
Base deficit >4 mEq/L
Fluid sequestration >6 L

WBC, white blood cell; LDH, lactate dehydrogenase; AST, aspartate aminotransferase; BUN, blood urea nitrogen; PaO_2, arterial oxygen tension.

Adapted from Banks PA. Am J Gastroenterol. 1997.

- A blunted PTH response to hypocalcemia

In this patient, the PTH level was 13 pg/mL. Even though this value is within normal range (11 to 54 pg/mL), it was considered relatively low because of the concurrent presence of hypocalcemia.

Why is hypoparathyroidism present? Because the hypocalcemia developed rapidly, reversible hypoparathyroidism is the most likely cause. Normal magnesium levels are necessary for both PTH release and the hormone's peripheral action. Hypomagnesemia is common in patients who require hospital admission for severe alcoholism. Others at risk for hypomagnesemia include patients with diabetes, those receiving diuretic therapy, and those with diarrhea.

Magnesium replacement therapy was instituted immediately after the calcium infusion was started (Table 8-2). It is important that neither treatment be delayed. A 2 g dose of magnesium sulfate (22 mg or 4 mL of 50% magnesium sulfate in a 100 mL solution) was delivered intravenously over 10 minutes, followed by a continuous infusion over the next 6 hours of 5 g diluted in saline or 5% dextrose in water. Hypomag-

Table 8-2. Boosting Magnesium Levels

When low serum magnesium levels prompt consideration of replacement therapy, the patient's condition determines the best route of administration. Oral therapy is generally preferred; the intravenous route is usually reserved for the patient who has significant cardiac or neuromuscular complications. Because serum magnesium is excreted renally, caution is warranted when administering magnesium replacement therapy to a patient who has decreased renal function.

Oral therapy

• Administer a 400 mg tablet of magnesium oxide four to six times daily. Each tablet contains about 20 mEq of elemental magnesium.

• Alternatively, consider administering magnesium sulfate or magnesium gluconate (either is less likely to cause diarrhea than magnesium oxide).

• Maintain the regimen for 3 or 4 days, regardless of the measured serum magnesium values, to build the body stores.

Intravenous therapy

• Initiate therapy with 2 g of magnesium sulfate (22 mgs or 4 mL of 50% magnesium sulfate in a 100 mL solution) infused over 10 minutes. Over the next 6 hours, administer a continuous infusion (5 g of magnesium sulfate diluted in saline or in 5% dextrose in water).

• Alternatively, consider the "Flink regimen." Administer a loading dose (6 g of magnesium sulfate in 1,000 mL of 5% dextrose in water) over 3 hours, followed by continuous infusions of magnesium sulfate (10 g in 2,000 mL of 5% dextrose in water over the next 24 hours, and then 6 g/d diluted from a 10% or 20% solution for the next 3 days).

nesemia should be treated regardless of the serum PTH level, especially when it accompanies hypocalcemia.

The patient's course was protracted despite the correction of his calcium and magnesium levels. A CT scan revealed necrotizing pancreatitis.

CASE 8-2. A 75-year-old Woman with Hypertension

A 75-year-old woman with chronic hypertension presented with nephrosclerosis. On admission, her blood pressure was 160/100 mm Hg. Laboratory findings included BUN, 48 mg/dL; creatinine, 4.2 mg/dL; sodium, 140 mEq/L; potassium, 5 mEq/L; chloride, 110 mEq/L; bicarbonate, 20 mEq/L; calcium, 8 mg/dL; and phosphorus, 5.2 mg/dL.

Albumin, globulin, and magnesium levels were normal. Urinalysis revealed only trace protein and no sediment. Renal ultrasonography demonstrated a symmetric decline in kidney size.

Table 8-3. Clinical conclusions for managing hypocalcemia

1 When your patient's total serum calcium level drops below 8.9 mg/dL, measure the serum level of ionized calcium or adjust the total serum calcium value for changes in serum protein concentrations to determine whether the hypocalcemia is real. The presence of Chvostek's sign and/or Trousseau's sign indicates there is neuromuscular irritability and supports a diagnosis of true hypocalcemia.

2 Institute emergent treatment if complications of hypocalcemia (such as tetany, neuromuscular irritability, hypotension, seizures, and ECG abnormalities) are evident. Administer elemental calcium (10 to 30 mL of 10% gluconate) diluted in 150 mL of 5% dextrose in water intravenously over approximately 10 minutes. More rapid infusions may lead to bradycardia and asystole. If the hypocalcemia persists, administer a continuous infusion of calcium gluconate at a rate of 0.3 to 2 mg/kg/h.

3 Be aware that hypomagnesemia commonly accompanies — and may even cause — hypocalcemia. Also, measure the patient's parathyroid hormone (PTH) levels. Reduced PTH levels or a weakening of the hormone's effectiveness can cause hypocalcemia, as can impaired conversion of vitamin D to its activated form.

4 If hypomagnesemia is present, initiate intravenous magnesium replacement therapy. Hypomagnesemia should be treated regardless of the PTH level.

5 Manage physiologic hypocalcemia with oral calcium carbonate supplements and, if needed, vitamin D supplements.

The patient was given an angiotensin-converting enzyme inhibitor to treat her hypertension; subsequently, her blood pressure dropped to 140/88 mm Hg. She had no complaints referable to her hypocalcemia; Chvostek's and Trousseau's signs were absent.

Is the hypocalcemia real? Because symptoms and signs of end-organ dysfunction due to hypocalcemia were absent and because the albumin level was normal, the problem was likely physiologic hypocalcemia. The PTH level was measured and found to be elevated (92 pg/mL). The combination of hypocalcemia, chronic renal failure, and an elevated PTH level pointed to a low level of activated vitamin D. The underlying cause was presumed to be decreased 1-hydroxylation, one of the two steps in the conversion of inactive vitamin D into its active form. Under such clinical circumstances (renal insufficiency), measurement of the serum vitamin D level was not necessary.

What treatment was required? The patient was treated with oral calcium supplements (2 calcium carbonate tablets with meals). She was also given vitamin D replacement therapy with calcitriol (a synthetic vitamin D analog), 0.25 mg/d orally.

The calcium carbonate not only increased her serum calcium level but also eliminated excess ingested phosphorus by binding it in the intestine. Elevated levels of plasma phosphorus further decreased calcium levels and stimulated PTH. The patient's serum calcium level rose to a value within the normal range; her PTH level decreased.

Suggested Reading

1. Banks PA. Practice guidelines in acute pancreatitis. *Am J Gastroenterol.* 1997;92:377-386.

2. Felsenfeld AJ. Considerations for the treatment of secondary hyperparathyroidism in renal failure. *J Am Soc Nephrol.* 1997;8:993-1004.

3. Flink EB. Magnesium deficiency. Etiology and clinical spectrum. *Acta Med Scand Suppl.* 1981;647:125-137.

4. Reber PM, Heath H III. Hypocalcemic emergencies. *Med Clin North Am.* 1995;79:93-106.

5. Trehan S, Rutecki GW, Whittier FC. Magnesium disorders: what to do when homeostasis goes awry. *Consultant.* 1996;36:2485-2497.

9. Hypercalcemia
The "3-hormone, 3-organ rule"

Calcium is essential to normal physiologic function in many organ systems. Muscle contraction, neuronal conduction, bone strength and integrity, enzyme activity, and the coagulation cascade all rely on calcium. Serum calcium levels must be regulated within a narrow range. The clinical consequences of severe calcium imbalance can be life-threatening. Hypercalcemia, which most often results from malignancy or hyperparathyroidism, can lead to mental obtundation, heart block, and cardiac arrest. Hypocalcemia is associated with neuromuscular irritability but may culminate in tetany and seizures.

Calcium Homeostasis

The clinical evaluation of calcium abnormalities may seem more complicated than that of other electrolyte disorders, primarily for two reasons:

- Electrolyte physiology often focuses on disparities between intracellular and extracellular concentrations. For example, the resting membrane potential depends on the difference between the intracellular and extracellular concentrations of potassium. Calcium activity, however, is unique in that it relies on the difference between its concentration in bone and in extracellular fluid. In the latter, calcium is mainly distributed as protein-bound, complexed, and ionized fractions. (The proportional distributions are 40%, 13%, and 47%, respectively.) The concentration of calcium relevant to health and disease is the serum ionized fraction.

- Also, calcium is an atypical electrolyte because its levels are delicately maintained by the "three-hormone, three-organ rule." Whereas levels of other electrolytes are regulated by one or two hormones or end-organs, calcium levels are governed by an ongoing, coordinated interplay among parathyroid hormone (PTH), activated vitamin D, and calcitonin (three regulatory hormones) with bone, kidney, and small intestine (three target organs). The regulatory pathways of calcium metabolism are shown in Figure 9-1.

Target Organs

Here we focus on the role of the small intestine and the kidney in calcium homeostasis. The contribution of bone (another important target organ) is included in our discussion of the regulatory hormones.

- **Small intestine.** The diet of a typical adult in this country contains roughly 1 g/d of calcium. Of that amount, approximately 400 mg is absorbed in the small intestine. Of the absorbed calcium, about 200 mg is then excreted into the bile and other intestinal secretions. Therefore, only 200 mg of the total amount of calcium ingested daily is available to circulate between bone and extracellular fluid. A deficient daily dietary intake of calcium results in increased intestinal absorption of calcium; however, if the intake is excessive, intestinal absorption decreases.

- **Kidney.** This organ is critical to the maintenance of calcium balance. The glomerulus filters out the calcium that is not bound to protein; this calcium is then handled differently by the separate nephron segments.

In the proximal tubule, approximately 50% to 70% of the filtered calcium is reabsorbed; there, calcium reabsorption mirrors sodium reabsorption. During volume expansion, increased sodium excretion correlates with increased calcium excretion. In volume-contracted states, increased sodium reabsorption correlates with increased calcium reabsorption.

The nephron segments between the proximal and distal tubules that contain the ascending limb of the loop of Henle reabsorb 30% to 40% of the filtered calcium. In the distal nephron, which reabsorbs about 10% of the filtered calcium, there is less of a link between volume and the reabsorption or excretion of sodium and calcium. Also, it is in this portion of the nephron that PTH and activated vitamin D (1,25-dihydroxyvitamin D) increase calcium reabsorption during calcium-deficient states.

Normally, the kidney excretes approximately 200 mg/d of calcium to maintain homeostasis. In patients with a calcium surplus, however, calcium excretion increases; in those with a calcium deficiency, it decreases. During states of severe calcium depletion, the kidney can decrease urinary calcium excretion to 50 mg/d or less.

This brief review of what happens to calcium in the renal tubules helps clarify how various groups of diuretics affect calcium balance. For example, loop diuretics affect tubular transport in the thick ascending limb of the loop of Henle and thereby increase the excretion of calcium.

Box 9-1. Technologic advances have changed options for hyperparathyroidism

Hyperparathyroidism has traditionally been described as a disease of "stones, bones, groans, and moans." Before the era of automated screening, asymptomatic hyperparathyroidism remained hidden until severe hypercalcemia became evident. Renal lithiasis from hypercalciuria (stones), osteitis fibrosa cystica (bones), pancreatitis and constipation (groans), and psychiatric abnormalities (moans) were the initial manifestations of what, by then, was a far-advanced disease.

Today, clinicians rarely see the end-stage of primary hyperparathyroidism. Instead, the condition may be uncovered when elevations in serum calcium levels are minimal. Patients with serum calcium readings below 11 mg/dL are usually asymptomatic and have mild to moderate elevations of parathyroid hormone.

The current management dilemma is one of timing: when should an adenoma be surgically removed to prevent serious eventual complications? An NIH Consensus Development Conference recommended parathyroidectomy in the following settings:
- A serum calcium level greater than 12 mg/dL
- Hypercalciuria greater than 400 mg/d
- The presence of symptoms and signs referable to parathyroid hormone excess — stones, bones, groans, or moans
- Markedly reduced cortical bone density
- Hypercalcemia causing a decreased glomerular filtration rate
- Patient age under 50 years

More recently, vertebral osteopenia has become a possible indication for surgery in patients with hyperparathyroidism. Patients with hyperparathyroidism and lumbar spine bone mineral density measurements greater than 1.5 standard deviations below the mean for age- and sex-matched controls actually gained bone mass (15% ± 3%) 1 year after parathyroidectomy, compared with a similar group followed medically. Furthermore, in postmenopausal women with mild primary hyperparathyroidism, estrogen replacement therapy can maintain bone mineral density, precluding the need for surgery.

In contrast, thiazides reduce urinary calcium excretion by exerting a direct effect on the distal tubules. In addition, this class of diuretics can cause volume contraction and thereby increase proximal tubular sodium and calcium reabsorption. Therefore, thiazide therapy may unmask hypercalcemia in those patients who have another subclinical abnormality in calcium metabolism (eg, early hyperparathyroidism).

It is also worth noting that in the distal convoluted tubule (DCT), a clear inverse relationship is seen between sodium and calcium reabsorption. This is the basis for using thiazide diuretics in patients who have hypercalciuric renal stones. The underlying mechanism depends not only on thiazide-induced volume depletion but also on the direct effects of thiazides on the tubules themselves. The recent discovery that inactivating mutations in the thiazide-sensitive Na-Cl cotransporter in the DCT reduce urinary calcium excretion, whereas inactivating mutations in the Na^+-K^+-2Cl cotransporter in the thick ascending limb produce hypercalciuria (despite volume depletion), supports this inverse relationship.

Regulatory Hormones

- **PTH.** An 84-amino-acid protein synthesized and released from the parathyroid gland in response to hypocalcemia, PTH increases the serum calcium concentration by its actions on the three target organs. It mobilizes calcium from bone by increasing osteoclast numbers and action, increases calcium reabsorption in the distal nephron, and stimulates the synthesis of 1,25-dihydroxyvitamin D. In turn, activated vitamin D elevates the intestinal absorption of calcium.

- **Activated vitamin D.** Originating from a precursor molecule, vitamin D requires two separate hydroxylations before it achieves full biologic potency. It must be metabolized to 25-hydroxyvitamin D in the liver and then further metabolized in the kidney to 1,25-dihydroxycholecalciferol, its active form. Activated vitamin D acts on the intestine to increase calcium absorption, on bone to increase calcium mobilization, and on the kidney to increase reabsorption within the distal tubule. In patients with renal disease, the important 1-hydroxylation is decreased; thus, the amount of active hormone available and its action on calcium metabolism also are decreased.

- **Calcitonin.** This 32-amino-acid polypeptide is made and released by the parafollicular cells of the thyroid gland in response to hypercalcemia. Calcitonin lowers serum levels of calcium by decreasing osteoclast activity and by stimulating a distal tubular-mediated calciuresis.

Calcium Imbalance

How to recognize. Most abnormalities in calcium metabolism are detected through the routine measurement of electrolyte levels via automated screening tests. However, such automated panels measure total serum levels of calcium, whether protein-bound, complexed, or ionized. As noted previously, the physiologically relevant serum calcium concentration is that of the ionized fraction. To determine this, either a specialized test should be ordered or an appropriate adjustment should

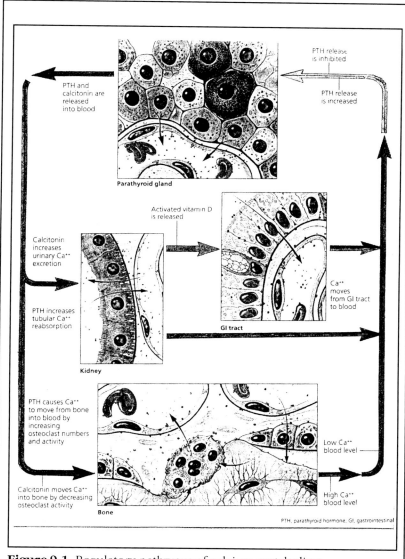

PTH release
is inhibited

PTH and
calcitonin are
released
into blood

PTH release
is increased

Parathyroid gland

Activated vitamin D
is released

Calcitonin
increases
urinary Ca⁺⁺
excretion

Ca⁺⁺
moves
from GI tract
to blood

PTH increases
tubular Ca⁺⁺
reabsorption

GI tract

Kidney

PTH causes Ca⁺⁺
to move from bone
into blood by
increasing
osteoclast numbers
and activity

Low Ca⁺⁺
blood level

Calcitonin moves Ca⁺⁺
into bone by decreasing
osteoclast activity

High Ca⁺⁺
blood level

Bone

PTH, parathyroid hormone, GI, gastrointestinal

Figure 9-1. Regulatory pathways of calcium metabolism

be made for changes in serum protein concentrations.

To make this adjustment, you should keep in mind that 40% of serum calcium is bound to protein. A 1 g/dL decrease in the serum albumin level reflects a 0.8 mg/dL decrease in the serum calcium level. (An equivalent change in serum globulins, either up or down, affects calcium concentrations by a lesser magnitude — 0.16 mg/dL. Thus, if a patient's serum albumin level drops from 4 to 2 mg/dL and the serum calcium level was previously measured at 9.2 mg/dL (within the normal range of 8.9 to 10.6 mg/dL), the calcium level should be expected to drop, according to the following calculation:

$$9.2 \text{ mg/dL} - (0.8 \times 2) = 7.6 \text{ mg/dL}$$

However, because this decrease represents a decline in protein-bound calcium and not a change in the ionized fraction, it has no adverse effects on normal physiology.

One additional factor that may alter the ionized calcium level is systemic pH. Alkalemia shifts hydrogen ions from plasma proteins to serum in an attempt to buffer the increase in bicarbonate. More of the ionized fraction of calcium will then be protein-bound by the "excess" negative charges left on plasma proteins. The opposite occurs with acidemia. Thus, hyperventilation with alkalemia may precipitate tetany in a patient with borderline hypocalcemia.

Which hormones to measure. Serum levels of the three calcium-related hormones can be determined by laboratory assays. The most essential measurement is that of PTH (Box 9-2). Recently developed immunometric assays recognize the intact PTH molecule by using two antibodies with specificity for two separate sites. Primary hyperparathyroidism is a common cause of hypercalcemia (Box 9-1).

Although both vitamin D and calcitonin levels also can be measured, the clinical usefulness of these values is less important than that of PTH. Vitamin D levels may be helpful in diagnosing diseases in which increased vitamin D synthesis and sensitivity to its action are responsible for hypercalcemia, such as sarcoidosis.

Case 9-1. A 66-year-old Woman with Lung Cancer

Our algorithm for diagnosing hypercalcemia is shown in Figure 9-2. To illustrate how this algorithm can be applied, we present a case in which a 66-year-old woman with a history of lung cancer was admitted for obtundation, nausea, vomiting, and polyuria.

The patient had recently lost 15 lb. She had a 50 pack/y smoking history and documented obstructive pulmonary disease ([FEV$_1$], 1.1 L; FEV$_1$ to forced vital capacity ratio, 30%). Unresectable squamous cell carcinoma of the lung, stage IIIB (T$_4$N$_1$M$_0$), had been diagnosed 6 months earlier.

The patient was difficult to arouse during examination, but manifestations of a focal neurologic deficit were absent. Her vital signs included: blood pressure, 100/50 mm Hg; pulse, 120 beats per minute and

Box 9-2. What the parathyroid hormone level reveals

The parathyroid hormone (PTH) level can be a clue to a number of underlying disorders. The listing below is not meant to be all-inclusive, but rather offers several possibilities when PTH is at a normal or increased level or when its level has dropped below the normal range.

Normal or increased PTH level

- Renal insufficiency is the most common cause and is associated with decreased 1-hydroxylation of vitamin D.
- If the vitamin D level is below normal and if the patient does not have renal disease, the problem may be fat malabsorption or severe hepatobiliary disease.
- Barbiturates, primidone, and phenytoin may decrease the level of active vitamin D.
- Pseudohypoparathyroidism or end-organ resistance to PTH action may be the problem, and subset designations have been established according to the cyclic adenosine monophosphate (cAMP) response to infused PTH. In type I, the infusion of PTH does not increase urinary cAMP; in type II, the infusion does have this effect. A characteristic physiognomy is present, and the diagnosis is made in childhood.

Decreased PTH level

Reversible problems
- A magnesium deficiency may be present.
- Surgery for parathyroid adenoma or hyperplasia or removal of a large thyroid malignancy decreases PTH; the same can occur, rarely, after ^{131}I irradiation for hyperthyroidism.

Irreversible problems
- The manufacture of PTH stops after surgical parathyroidectomy.
- Congenital hypoparathyroidism is inherited as an autosomal dominant, G-protein receptor mutation; it may also be X-linked, or autosomal recessive.

Developmental problems
- DiGeorge syndrome and other rare diseases, such as Kenney-Caffey syndrome, may be involved.

Autoimmune problems
- Low PTH levels occur with mucocutaneous candidiasis and hypoadrenalism, which is autosomal recessive.
- An autoimmune basis for low PTH levels is diagnosed in childhood.

regular; respirations, 24 breaths per minute; and temperature, 36.7°C (98°F). Initial laboratory findings included: sodium, 138 mEq/L; potassium, 4.8 mEq/L; chloride, 106 mEq/L; bicarbonate, 21 mEq/L; BUN, 30 mg/dL; creatinine, 1.6 mg/dL; albumin, 2.8 mg/dL; calcium, 13.6 mg/dL; phosphorus, 2 mg/dL.

How serious is the hypercalcemia? As the diagnostic algorithm shows, this patient's hypercalcemia is quite serious. The absolute value of measured calcium was high. When corrected for the 1.2 mg/dL drop in the serum albumin level (from 4.0 to 2.8 mg/dL), the total calcium level should have declined by about 1 mg/dL ([0.8 x 1.2] = 0.96 mg/dL). Instead, the corrected value was 14.8 mg/dL (13.6 + 1.2). In addition, the patient has symptoms and signs (obtundation) of the calcium elevation. The degree of hypercalcemia and the accompanying symptoms indicated that the patient was in a hypercalcemic crisis; immediate treatment was required.

What are the treatment options? The three most frequently recommended approaches to the treatment of hypercalcemia include:

- Increasing the renal excretion of calcium by inducing volume expansion and then (possibly) by administering a loop diuretic

- Inhibiting bone reabsorption

- Initiating dialysis if the hypercalcemia is extreme — that is, complicated by marked volume contraction and renal failure

All hypercalcemic patients are volume-contracted. The mechanisms leading to volume loss include nephrogenic diabetes insipidus from hypercalcemia; decreased oral intake complicated by nausea and vomiting; and, in some patients, the concurrent use of thiazides, which increase renal tubular calcium reabsorption.

Therapeutic agents for hypercalcemia include the bisphosphonates, calcitonin, mithramycin, and gallium nitrate. The bisphosphonates, which inhibit osteoclast function, are the most frequently used. The most potent is pamidronate; this agent may be administered as a 60 to 90 mg IV infusion over 24 hours. In clinical trials, 70% to 100% of patients had decreased serum calcium levels within 24 hours of treatment, and as many as two-thirds of this group demonstrated normalized serum calcium levels within seven days. However, because bisphosphonates are excreted by the kidney, the dosage must be adjusted for those patients who have impaired kidney function.

Calcitonin is not as effective as the bisphosphonates. Calcitonin does lower calcium levels, but tachyphylaxis quickly occurs and limits therapeutic efficacy. Toxic effects limit use of the chemotherapeutic agent mithramycin. This drug is reserved for difficult cases of hypercalcemia that are related to malignancy. Gallium nitrate is not used as frequently

Figure 9-2. Hypercalcemia: A diagnostic algorithm

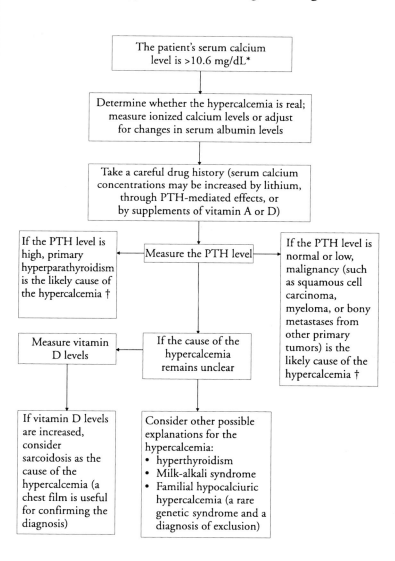

*Emergency treatment is indicated for patients with moderate hypercalcemia (serum calcium levels, 12 to 13.9 mg/dL) or severe hypercalcemia (serum calcium levels, >14 mg/dL) who have evidence of volume contraction and/or obtundation.

†Between 80% and 90% of all hypercalcemias are caused by either malignancy or hyperparathyroidism.4,10

Clinical Conclusions:

Diagnosing and managing hypercalcemia

1 Most cases of hypercalcemia are caused by primary hyperparathyroidism or a malignancy. In the absence of these conditions, sarcoidosis, hyperthyroidism, milk-alkali syndrome, and familial hypocalciuric hypercalcemia are possibilities.

2 The three organs involved in regulating serum calcium levels are the kidney, bone, and small intestine. The three hormones that are also key to calcium homeostasis are parathyroid hormone, activated vitamin D, and calcitonin.

3 If hypercalcemia is suspected based on the routine automated screening of electrolytes, it is essential to identify the level of the ionized fraction of serum calcium to determine how severe the patient's condition is and whether emergent treatment is needed.

4 Renal excretion of calcium can be increased by the induction of volume expansion — and possibly by the administration of a loop diuretic.

5 Inhibiting the bone release of calcium is another treatment option. The bisphosphonates are most often used for this purpose.

6 Corticosteroids can be useful for selected hypercalcemic patients. These drugs lower the intestinal absorption of calcium and seem to be most effective when the underlying problem is myeloma, lymphoma, sarcoidosis, or vitamin D toxicity.

---

as the bisphosphonates. The need to infuse it over five days and its potential for causing nephrotoxicity limit its usefulness.

Corticosteroids are effective for the hypercalcemia caused by myeloma, lymphoma, sarcoidosis, or vitamin D toxicity because they decrease the intestinal absorption of calcium. A dose of 200 to 300 mg of hydrocortisone or its equivalent is given daily for up to 5 days. Unfortunately, the response is slow, which limits the use of corticosteroids for patients in a hypercalcemic crisis.

Hemodialysis against a zero- or low-calcium bath may be used in selected circumstances to manage severe hypercalcemia. One such setting is hypercalcemia complicated by renal failure. Because the bisphosphonates and gallium nitrate are excreted by the kidney — and because corticosteroids and calcitonin are not immediately effective — dialysis may be lifesaving. Also, renal failure may preclude volume loading with normal saline.

How was therapy implemented? Vigorous volume expansion

with normal saline (approximately 200 mL/h) was initiated. The patient was reexamined frequently to ensure adequate volume repletion and to prevent volume overload. Only after volume had been restored adequately was a loop diuretic (furosemide, 20 to 40 mg IV q4 to 6h) administered to enhance calciuresis.

The patient's mental status subsequently improved, her blood pressure rose to 120/80 mm Hg, her BUN level decreased to 20 mg/dL, her creatinine level dropped to 1.2 mg/dL, and her serum calcium level dropped to 12.4 mg/dL.

The next intervention was targeted to inhibit the bone release of calcium. The patient was given pamidronate.

What was the outcome? This woman's PTH level was low (20 pg/ mL). Bony metastases were absent. Squamous cell cancers produce a PTH-related peptide (PTHrP) that activates the PTH receptor in a manner similar to native PTH. Even though PTHrP is larger than PTH, its homology with the parent hormone allows it to bind to the target receptor. Life expectancy in patients with cancer-associated hypercalcemia is poor. This patient died 3 months after this episode despite normalization of calcium levels.

Suggested Reading

1. Adams JS, Diz MM, Sharma OP. Effective reduction in the serum 1,25 dihydroxyvitamin D and calcium concentration in sarcoidosis-associated hypercalcemia with short-course chloroquine therapy. *Ann Intern Med.* 1989;111:437-438.
2. Edelson GW, Kleenehoper M. Hypercalcemic crisis. *Med Clin North Am.* 1995;79:79-92.
3. Grey AB, Stapleton JP, Evans MC, et al. Effect of hormone replacement therapy on bone mineral density in post-menopausal women with mild primary hyperparathyroidism. *Ann Intern Med.* 1996;125:360-368.
4. Leehey PS, Ing TS. Correction of hypercalcemia and hypophosphatemia by hemodialysis using a conventional, calcium-containing dialysis solution enriched with phosphorus. *Am J Kidney Dis.* 1997;29:288-290.
5. Mallette LE. The hypercalcemias. *Semin Nephrol.* 1992;12:159-190.
6. Muldowney WP, Mazbar SA. Rolaids-yogurt syndrome: a 1990s version of milk-alkali syndrome. *Am J Kidney Dis.* 1996;27:270-272.
7. Pearce SHS, Williamson C, Kifor O, et al. A familial syndrome of hypocalcemia with hypercalciuria due to mutations in the calcium-sensing receptor. *N Engl J Med.* 1996;335:1115-1122.
8. Potts JT. Hyperparathyroidism and other hypercalcemic disorders. *Ann Intern Med.* 1996;41:165-212.

9. Potts JT, ed. 1991 NIH Consensus Development Conference Statement on Primary Hyperparathyroidism. *J Bone Miner Res.* 1991;6:S9-S13.

10. Ralston SH, Gallacher SJ, Patel U, et al. Cancer-associated hypercalcemia: morbidity and mortality — clinical experience in 126 treated patients. *Ann Intern Med.* 1990;112:499-504.

11. Ratcliffe WA, Hutchesson ACJ, Bundred NJ, et al. Role of assays for parathyroid-hormone-related protein in investigation of hypercalcemia. *Lancet.* 1992;339:164-167.

12. Silverberg SJ, Locker FG, Bilezikian JP. Vertebral osteopenia: a new indication for surgery in primary hyperparathyroidism. *J Clin Endocrinol Metab.* 1996;81:4007-4012.

13. Warrell RP Jr, Murphy WK, Schulman P, et al. A randomized double-blind study of gallium nitrate compared with etidronate for acute control of cancer-related hypercalcemia. *J Clin Oncol.* 1991;9:1467-1475.

10. Phosphate Imbalance
When to Suspect, How to Treat

Phosphate imbalance is common among critically ill patients. It can result either from the illness itself or from its treatment. Phosphate imbalance also can lead to the development of respiratory or cardiac arrest as well as other adverse events.

Phosphate depletion, for example, can result from respiratory alkalemia and uncontrolled diabetes mellitus. Phosphate wasting also has been associated with disorders that affect the proximal tubules of the kidney (such as drug toxicity, multiple myeloma, and amyloidosis) as well as with malabsorption, alcoholism, and vitamin D deficiency. Iatrogenic causes of hypophosphatemia include hyperalimentation and the use of feeding formulas that contain an inadequate amount of phosphorus; in addition, volume expansion and diuretic therapy can impair phosphate resorption.

Hyperphosphatemia is seen less often then hypophosphatemia. Renal insufficiency is usually responsible, but hyperphosphatemia also can result from the intracellular release of phosphate stores (as occurs with the lysis of red blood cells, skeletal muscle, or tumor cells).

The consequences of phosphate imbalance can be severe. Phosphate is a key ion in the energy transfer process. Thus, hypophosphatemia can lead to muscle weakness and thereby to respiratory failure, congestive cardiomyopathy, rhabdomyolysis, and/or cardiac arrest. Occasionally, hypophosphatemia results in depressed chemotaxis and phagocytosis by white blood cells (increasing the risk of life-threatening infection) or in platelet dysfunction (increasing the risk of bleeding). Although the effects of hyperphosphatemia tend to be less serious, it can cause severe hypocalcemia, which can lead to tetany and cardiac arrhythmias.

Hypophosphatemia

What causes the imbalance? Too often, phosphate depletion is neither well understood nor readily recognized in clinical practice. The first appreciation of phosphate depletion as a cause of critical illness occurred at the end of World War II. During the liberation of concentration camps, soldiers often gave candy bars to camp survivors, who were already phosphate-deficient because of malnutrition. In many, the consumption of glucose led to severe phosphate depletion (a critical component of nutritional recovery syndrome), followed by respiratory arrest and death.

Once the link between glucose administration and severe hypophosphatemia was recognized, the administration of powdered milk (which contains phosphate but no glucose) to persons at high risk for hypophosphatemia during nutritional recovery was recommended. The incidence of respiratory arrest and sudden death among this population subsequently declined.

Hypophosphatemia is defined as a serum phosphate level below 2.5 mg/dL. It is generally attributed to one of three mechanisms:

- Decreased intestinal absorption
- Excessive urinary losses
- Transcellular shifts of the phosphate ion

However, in any single patient, two or more of these factors may be present. Less than 1% of total body phosphorus content is extracellular; therefore, shifts of phosphate into the cells can produce striking hypophosphatemia.

The causes of hypophosphatemia are listed in Table 10-1. Mild to moderate hypophosphatemia rarely produces signs and symptoms. It is only when the phosphate level is below 1 mg/dL that adverse effects become evident. Muscle weakness and myalgias are the earliest indications of severe depletion and may be followed by the development of

Table 10-1. Causes of hypophosphatemia

Mild to moderate (serum phosphate level, 1-2.5 mg/dL)
Asthma
Chronic obstructive pulmonary disease
Dialysis
Diuretic therapy
Glucose infusion
Hyperparathyroidism
Insulin administration
Kidney transplantation
Malabsorption
Renal tubular loss (Fanconi's syndrome)
Vitamin D deficiency
Volume expansion*

Severe (serum phosphate level, <1 mg/dL)
Chronic alcoholism
Chronic respiratory alkalosis
Diabetic ketoacidosis[†]
Excessive use of phosphate binders
Hyperalimentation
Nutritional recovery syndrome
Severe burns

*Moderately severe hypophosphatemia may result from hyperaldosteronism and during volume expansion with saline infusion.
[†]Severe hypophosphatemia may occur during the treatment of diabetic ketoacidosis.

respiratory arrest and congestive heart failure. The biochemical processes underlying these findings are complex, but two merit special mention.

The first process involves the phosphorylation of glucose and the formation of adenosine triphosphate during glycolysis. Because circulating phosphate is the direct source for the needed phosphorus, the energy transfer derived from glycolysis is prevented when the phosphate deficiency is severe. The lack of energy contributes to muscle weakness and muscle fatigue. If this persists, rhabdomyolysis may be a direct result.

The second biochemical process involves a reduction in 2,3-diphosphoglycerate in red blood cells that occurs when the serum concentration of phosphorus decreases and hemoglobin's affinity for oxygen increases. This creates a lack of oxygen release and is followed by an increase in cardiac output. The resulting combination of a reduced oxygen release, elevated cardiac output, and cardiac muscle weakness may lead to the simultaneous failure of respiratory and cardiac muscles.

Which patients are at risk? Severe hypophosphatemia can develop in patients with severe burn injury for a number of reasons:

- Tissue regeneration requires tremendous phosphate repletion.

- These patients hyperventilate, causing phosphate to shift into cells.

- Volume repletion and renal tubular injury result in a phosphate diuresis.

Hypophosphatemia may also be present in patients undergoing dialysis when phosphate binders are instrumental in management. The administration of glucose during hyperalimentation is a common cause of hypophosphatemia in critically ill patients (as was the candy consumption by concentration camp survivors). For this reason, adequate phosphate must be included in enteral and parenteral feeding formulas.

Two groups of patients are at particularly high risk for severe hypophosphatemia — those who have chronic alcoholism and those who are receiving therapy for diabetic ketoacidosis.

Chronic alcoholism. Phosphate depletion occurs in as many as 50% of patients with chronic alcoholism. Factors that may contribute to the low phosphate level in these patients include poor diet, diarrhea, and vomiting. Long-term alcohol abusers also experience an excessive urinary loss of phosphate and the renal wasting of uric acid. This is thought to result from alcohol's direct effect on the reabsorption of phosphate and uric acid in the renal tubule.

To further complicate matters, the onset of alcoholic cirrhosis may be accompanied by the development of respiratory alkalemia, which can become chronic. Respiratory alkalemia causes a decrease in the carbon dioxide tension, intracellular alkalemia, increased glycolysis, and a shift of phosphate into cells (Figure 10-1).

Case 10-1. A 41-year-old Man with Chronic Alcoholism

A 41-year-old man presented with a grand mal seizure. The medical history revealed long-term ethanol abuse. On physical examination, the patient was tremulous. His blood pressure was 140/100 mm Hg, and his pulse rate was 110 beats per minute. The liver edge was felt 3 cm below the right costal margin; intraosseous muscle wasting was also noted. A CT scan of the head was normal.

Laboratory findings. Admission laboratory values included: blood urea nitrogen, 10 mg/dL; serum creatinine, 1 mg/dL; serum sodium, 138 mEq/L; serum potassium, 3.9 mEq/L; serum chloride, 102 mEq/L; serum bicarbonate, 23 mEq/L; uric acid, 2.6 mg/dL; serum calcium, 8.2 mg/dL; serum phosphate, 2 mg/dL; albumin, 2.7 g/dL; bilirubin, 2.8 mg/dL; and serum magnesium, 1 mg/dL.

Early course. An infusion of 5% dextrose in half normal saline was initiated at a rate of 100 mL/h; thiamine (100 mg) was administered. After 24 hours, respiratory failure developed, and the patient was intubated. The pulmonary and cardiology services were consulted. On auscultation, a loud S_3 gallop and bibasilar rales were heard. The chest film findings were compatible with acute pulmonary edema.

Discussion. This case highlights several key points in the diagnosis and management of hypophosphatemia.

- **Since the serum phosphate level was mildly to moderately depressed on admission, what factor (or factors) may have precipitated the development of severe phosphate depletion?**

  Two possibilities would be the administration of intravenous glucose and the presence of cirrhosis, which resulted in respiratory alkalemia.

- **Can the patient's cardiac failure and pulmonary edema be related to severe hypophosphatemia?**

  Severe hypophosphatemia may cause cardiac failure in two ways. It can instigate a shift in the oxygen dissociation curve that results in oxygen deprivation to the heart. Also, it can inhibit glycolysis and thereby an important source of energy for the cardiac muscle.

- **Could intravenous phosphorus replacement therapy improve cardiac function?**

  Improvement in cardiac output following phosphate replacement has been demonstrated.

- **Diabetic ketoacidosis.** In patients with diabetic ketoacidosis, glycosuria, ketonuria, and osmotic diuresis lead to excessive phosphate loss in the urine. Initially, however, the phosphate level may be normal or near normal because with intracellular insulin deficiency the use of phosphate for energy production decreases. In addition, metabolic hetoacidemia causes phosphate to shift out of the cells. During insulin therapy, serum glucose levels decrease, and intracellular glucose metabolism increases; also, with the correction of the acidemia, phosphate shifts back into the cells. Although uncommon, the result can be severe hypophosphatemia.

CASE 10-2. A 30-year-old Woman with Diabetic Ketoacidosis

A 30-year-old woman with a 20-year history of insulin-dependent diabetes mellitus presented at the emergency department. She stopped

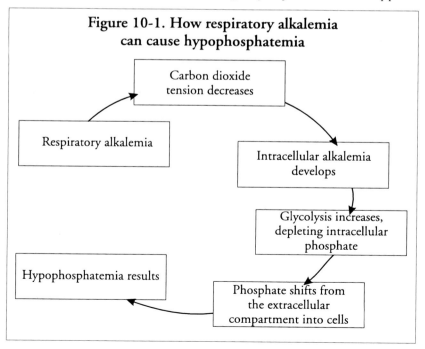

Figure 10-1. How respiratory alkalemia can cause hypophosphatemia

Respiratory alkalemia → Carbon dioxide tension decreases → Intracellular alkalemia develops → Glycolysis increases, depleting intracellular phosphate → Phosphate shifts from the extracellular compartment into cells → Hypophosphatemia results

Table 10-2. Phosphorus preparations

Preparation	Quantity containing 1 g of phosphorus
Oral	
Milk	Quart
Phospho-soda	6.2 mL
Neutra-Phos	300 mL or 4 capsules
Neutra-Phos-K	300 mL or 4 capsules
Phos-tabs	6 tablets
Intravenous	
In-Phos	40 mL
Hyper-phos-K	15 mL

taking her insulin 3 days earlier when symptoms of gastroenteritis developed. She complained of dizziness, polydipsia, and polyuria.

Physical findings included: blood pressure, 90/60 mm Hg; respiration rate, 28 breaths per minute; pulse rate 120 beats per minute; temperature 36.9°C (98.4°F). Other physical findings were normal.

Laboratory findings. Admission laboratory values included: blood urea nitrogen (BUN), 12 mg/dL; serum creatinine, 1 mg/dL; serum glucose, 1,050 mg/dL; serum sodium, 120 mEq/L; serum potassium, 5.7 mEq/L; serum chloride, 90 mEq/L; serum bicarbonate, 5 mEq/L; pH, 7.12; carbon dioxide tension, 13 mm Hg.

Early course. An insulin drip was initiated, and an infusion of 2 L of normal saline was given over the first 8 hours. The admission laboratory tests were repeated and revealed BUN, 10 mg/dL; serum creatinine, 1 mg/dL; serum glucose, 150 mg/dL; serum sodium, 135 mEq/L; serum potassium, 3.6 mEq/L; serum chloride, 95 mEq/L; serum bicarbonate, 12 mEq/L. Over the next 4 hours, glucose and potassium were added to the intravenous fluids. The patient reported progressive muscle weakness and shortness of breath.

Discussion. This case highlights the risks of hypophosphatemia associated with diabetes ketoacidosis.

- **What would you predict the serum phosphate level to be at the time of the muscle weakness?**

  The serum phosphate level would likely be below 1 mg/dL.

- **What factors contributed to the onset of the hypophos-**

phatemia in this patient?

First, the partial correction of metabolic acidemia encouraged a shift of phosphate into the cells. Second, the glucose transfer and utilization within the cells likely resulted in the removal of phosphate from the serum pool. Third, the administration of large amounts of intravenous fluids probably exacerbated the phosphate dilution.

- **How should treatment be initiated in this patient?**

Initially, potassium phosphate (5 mg/kg, diluted in half normal or normal saline) should be given intravenously over 6 to 8 hours. The patient's serum potassium and serum phosphate levels should then be obtained to guide further therapy.

How the imbalance is corrected. Hypophosphatemia, regardless of the underlying cause, is treated with oral or intravenous phosphorus replacement therapy. In a patient with chronic alcoholism, any degree of hypophosphatemia warrants prompt phosphorus replacement, usually with oral supplements or dairy products. However, when the serum phosphate level falls below 1.5 mg/dL, parenteral therapy may be indicated. In patients with diabetic ketoacidosis, potassium replacement is also required; thus, potassium phosphate salts are often used for initial therapy.

Dosage recommendations for phosphorus replacement are expressed in milligrams per kilogram or millimoles per kilogram for elemental phosphorus but only in millimoles per kilogram for the anion phosphate. Thirty-one milligrams of elemental phosphorus is equivalent to 1 mmol of phosphate.

Options for oral therapy include milk and phosphate salts (Table 10-2). One quart of skim milk or low-fat milk contains 1 g of phosphorus; milk is an ideal choice when gradual phosphorus replacement is required and the patient can tolerate oral therapy. Milk also can be supplemented with or replaced by oral phosphate salts. Initially, 1 to 2 g/d of phosphorus should be given in divided doses.

Intravenous replacement therapy is usually reserved for patients with severe hypophosphatemia (with serum phosphate levels at or below 1.5 mg/dL). A phosphate level of 1 mg/dL is a harbinger of the most serious complications of phosphate depletion. However, it may be best to consider parenteral therapy when phosphate levels are slightly above 1 mg/dL to prevent respiratory or cardiac arrest. Because parenteral preparations have been associated with serious side effects, they are reserved for the most serious clinical situations. Complications of intravenous phosphorus replacement therapy include:

- Acute renal failure

- Calcification of the bundle of His (resulting in heart block and sudden cardiac death)

- Hypocalcemia with tetany

- Hypomagnesemia

- Hyperphosphatemia

- Soft-tissue calcification

Phosphate distribution varies from one patient to another, and formulas have not been developed to predict the precise pretreatment deficit. The usual initial intravenous dose of elemental phosphorus is 2.5 to 5 mg/kg, administered over 6 to 8 hours.

Phosphate salts may be diluted in normal saline, half normal saline, or a solution of 5% dextrose in water. However, phosphate salts should not be added to lactated Ringer's solution; because it contains calcium, salts of calcium and phosphate will precipitate out. On the other hand, phosphate salts are more soluble in formulas for total parenteral nutrition that contain calcium; the amino acids in these formulas lower the pH of the solution. If the multiplication product of the formula's calcium concentration (in milliequivalents per milliliter) and the phosphorus concentration (in millimoles per milliliter) is below 200, calcium-phosphate precipitates usually will not form.

The response to phosphorus replacement therapy in any given patient cannot be predicted. Therefore, we strongly advise monitoring the serum phosphate level, obtaining measurements twice each day.

Hyperphosphatemia

What causes the imbalance? The most common cause of hyperphosphatemia is renal insufficiency. It is often seen in patients with renal failure (acute or chronic) but is most severe in those with acute renal failure secondary to rhabdomyolysis or with tumor lysis syndrome. Less common causes of hyperphosphatemia include malignant hyperthermia, thyrotoxicosis, hypoparathyroidism, and acromegaly. Hyperphosphatemia itself may produce no symptoms; thus, the diagnosis is usually made from routine electrolyte measurements.

The major complication of hyperphosphatemia is hypocalcemia. This is mediated by increased ionized calcium binding by the elevated phosphorus level and by a decrease in active vitamin D (1,25-

dihydroxyvitamin D). In patients with chronic hyperphosphatemia, metastatic calcification can occur because of the elevated product of calcium and phosphorus.

Because the complications of hyperphosphatemia are not as predictable as those associated with phosphate depletion, phosphate levels for mild, moderate, and severe disease are not usually specified. Acute and severe complications — especially hypocalcemia — are particularly likely to occur in patients with disorders such as tumor lysis syndrome complicated by acute renal insufficiency. In such situations, phosphate levels can exceed 15 mg/dL within a short time.

How the imbalance is corrected. Hyperphosphatemia is best treated by managing the underlying renal insufficiency to prevent the metabolic bone disease of uremia. Renal disease affects a number of electrolytes and hormones that are critical to bone metabolism. For example, a decrease in the glomerular filtration rate increases serum phosphate levels. This, in turn, decreases serum calcium levels and

---

Clinical conclusions.

Managing phosphate imbalance

1 Hypophosphatemia is caused by decreased intestinal absorption, excessive urinary losses, and/or transcellular shifts in distribution. Patients with chronic alcoholism or diabetic ketoacidosis are at high risk for a phosphate disorder.

2 Unless the phosphate depletion is severe, a patient is likely to be asymptomatic. However, when serum phosphate levels fall below 1 mg/dL, muscle weakness and myalgias become evident and may be followed by congestive heart failure, respiratory arrest, and/or cardiac arrest.

3 Oral phosphorus replacement therapy is preferred over intravenous therapy because it is less likely to be accompanied by serious side effects. However, intravenous therapy is recommended for patients with serum phosphate levels below 1.5 mg/dL.

4 Because the response to the phosphorus replacement therapy cannot be predicted, serum phosphate levels should be monitored during treatment.

5 Renal insufficiency is the most common cause of hyperphosphatemia; treatment of the phosphate imbalance is directed at correcting the renal dysfunction. Vigorous treatment (such as dialysis) is used for severe, acute hyperphosphatemia with renal failure (rhabdomyolysis), chronic or end-stage renal failure.

increases parathyroid hormone concentrations. All of these changes adversely affect bone. In addition, renal disease decreases active vitamin D synthesis in the kidney (the 1-hydroxylation of vitamin D), also negatively impacting the integrity of bone.

Because renal failure is almost invariably associated with hyperphosphatemia, two methods are used to treat phosphate excess. GI tract phosphate-binding antacids (for example, calcium carbonate or acetate) may be prescribed for patients who have chronic renal insufficiency. In those with acute hyperphosphatemia or end-stage renal failure, dialysis is used to lower the serum phosphate levels.

When hyperphosphatemia occurs in patients who have diseases that are not associated with renal failure (such as acromegaly), the serum phosphate levels are usually not high enough to be clinically significant. In such cases, treatment of the primary disease is recommended.

Suggested Reading

1.   Bollaert PE, Levy B, Nace L, et al. Hemodynamic and metabolic effects of rapid correction of hypophosphatemia in patients with septic shock. *Chest*. 1995;107:1698-1701.

2.   Fisher JN, Kitabchi AE. A randomized study of phosphate therapy in the treatment of diabetic ketoacidosis. *J Clin Endocrinol Metab*. 1983;57:177-180.

3.   Hoft SD, Rowlands BJ. Guillain-Barré syndrome due to hypophosphatemia following intravenous hyperalimentation. *JPEN*. 1988;12:414-416.

4.   Knochel JP. Hypophosphatemia in the alcoholic. *Arch Intern Med*. 1980;140:613-615.

5.   Lichtman MA, Miller DR, Cohen J, et al. Reduced red cell glycolysis, 2,3-diphosphoglycerate and adenosine triphosphate concentration and increased hemoglobin-oxygen affinity caused by hypophosphatemia. *Ann Intern Med*. 1971;74:562-568.

6.   Perreault MM, Ostrop NK, Tiemey MG. Efficacy and safety of intravenous phosphate replacement in critically ill patients. *Ann Pharmacother*. 1997;31:683-688.

7.   Rosen GH, Boullata JI, O'Rangers EA, et al. Intravenous phosphate repletion regimen for critically ill patients with moderate hypophosphatemia. *Crit Care Med*. 1995;23:1204-1210.

8.   Sacks GS, Walker J, Dickerson RN, et al. Observations of hypophosphatemia and its management in nutrition support. *Nutr Clin Pract*. 1994;9:105-108.

9.   Singhal PC, Kumar A, Desroches L, et al. Prevalence and predictors of rhabdomyolysis in patients with hypophosphatemia. *Am J Med*. 1982;92:458-464.

11. Magnesium Disorders
What to Do when Homeostasis Goes Awry

After potassium, magnesium is the second most common intracellular cation in the body. Within the cell, magnesium is ubiquitous; it is essential for the maintenance of energy homeostasis and is actively involved in every aspect of cellular metabolism. Magnesium plays a key role in oxidative phosphorylation through its presence in adenosine triphosphatase (ATPase), in anaerobic phosphorylation, in muscle function through creatinine kinase, and in the important cellular conductive functions of the calcium and potassium channels.

The maintenance of body magnesium stores within narrow limits is essential to cellular energy production. Depletion or excess of body magnesium stores may have profound effects on cardiovascular function. The normal range of serum magnesium is approximately 1.5 to 2.0 (± 0.2) mEq/L, which is maintained by the concomitant interplay of regulatory mechanisms that act mainly on the kidney, intestine, and bone. Healthy men require 350 mg/d; women need 300 mg/d.

Recently, magnesium imbalance has been implicated in several cardiovascular disorders, including ventricular arrhythmias, ischemic heart disease, and hypertension. In addition, the treatment of hypomagnesemia after cardiac surgery has been shown to markedly reduce ventricular dysrhythmias and overall morbidity. Alcoholic and diabetic persons and those taking diuretics, digitalis, or certain chemotherapeutic agents are at particularly high risk for magnesium deficiency.

Hypermagnesemia, though uncommon, may occur in persons who have decreased renal magnesium excretion. The disorder may be fatal if untreated.

Here we review causes, manifestations (and implications), and therapy for hypomagnesemia and hypermagnesemia. We offer four case studies to help you evaluate and treat disturbances in magnesium homeostasis.

Hypomagnesemia

Magnesium deficiency is quite common (Table 11-1). It occurs in up to 11% of hospitalized patients and 52% of patients in coronary care units.

Hypomagnesemia can be classified as acute or chronic. The most common diagnoses in patients with acute magnesium depletion are malignancy, chronic obstructive pulmonary disease, and alcoholism; coronary artery disease (CAD) and bypass surgery are also associated with acute magnesium deficiency.

Alcoholism, liver disease, diabetes mellitus, and carcinoma are most frequently associated with chronic hypomagnesemia. In fact, the incidence of hypomagnesemia is 25% to 39% among patients who have diabetes mellitus.

Types of hypomagnesemia and associated factors. The major types and causes of hypomagnesemia are shown in Table 11-1.

Alcoholism. As noted, low magnesium levels are frequently associated with acute and chronic alcoholism, as well as with alcohol withdrawal. In fact, some studies have demonstrated that all alcoholic patients who require hospital admission are magnesium-deficient to some degree. Several mechanisms may contribute to such depletion in alcoholics. These include decreased dietary intake and occasionally, coexisting chronic pancreatitis resulting in fat malabsorption and diarrhea.

Alcohol may also cause magnesium loss by a direct effect on the renal tubule. The deficit in magnesium stores may be worsened by secondary hyperaldosteronism and the use of diuretics to manage the ascites of alcoholic cirrhosis.

Drugs. A number of agents are also associated with hypo-magnesemia (Table11- 2). Diuretics affect magnesium reabsorption and excretion differently, depending on their site of action in the nephron. Between 20% and 30% of filtered magnesium is reabsorbed in the proximal portion of the nephron. (The increased urinary loss of magnesium associated with seldom-used proximal tubular diuretics [eg, carbonic anhydrase inhibitors] is consistent with this.)

However, most magnesium reabsorption (approximately two thirds) occurs in the thick ascending limb of the loop of Henle. Reabsorption is so efficient in these two segments that daily urinary magnesium excretion may decrease to less than 1 mEq/L in states of magnesium deficiency. Obviously, diuretics such as furosemide that work at the loop of Henle can cause substantial magnesuria and magnesium depletion.

Table 11-1. Types and causes of hypomagnesemia

Excessive renal losses of magnesium

Acute and chronic effects of alcohol ingestion

Gitelman's syndrome

Cyclosporine therapy in renal transplant patients

The diuretic phase of acute renal failure

Osmotic diuresis

Renal tubular defects

Use of diuretics or certain drugs with effects on the kidney (e.g., cisplatinum)

Inadequate intestinal absorption or loss of magnesium in the stool

Bowel resection

Chronic bowel disease

Chronic diarrhea (as might be seen in patients with AIDS)

Laxative abuse

Malabsorption syndromes

Inadequate dietary intake

Parenteral replacement with solutions deficient in magnesium

Starvation

Rarer conditions

Excessive losses of electrolytes with sweating (resembling redistribution hypokalemia)

"Hungry bone" syndrome

Intracellular magnesium redistribution (as might occur with insulin therapy)

Pancreatitis

In contrast, diuretic agents that have more distal action have a varied effect on magnesium excretion. Thiazides can cause significant long-term loss, whereas aldosterone antagonists can actually increase serum levels of magnesium.

Other agents can cause urinary magnesium wasting by direct tubular injury and loss of tubular cell membrane integrity. In fact, cisplatin-induced magnesium deficiency may become permanent even when the drug is discontinued.

Endocrine abnormalities. Several endocrine abnormalities may contribute to hypomagnesemia. Diabetic ketoacidosis and uncontrolled diabetes lead to magnesium deficiency, perhaps because of the osmotic diuresis and resultant decrease in proximal tubular reabsorption of magnesium. Hyperaldosteronism and hyperthyroidism have also been associated with hypomagnesemia, possibly secondary to volume expansion and increased filtration, respectively. Hypercalcemia is frequently associated with decreased levels of magnesium and elevated urinary calcium levels appear to inhibit magnesium reabsorption in the loop of Henle.

Table 11-2. Agents that may cause hypomagnesemia through renal loss
Aminoglycoside antibiotics
Amphotericin B
Cisplatin
Cyclosporine
Digoxin
Diuretics
Foscarnet
Pentamidine

Clinical manifestations. These occur predominantly in the heart and nervous system. Cardiac manifestations may include sudden cardiac death and an increased incidence of arrhythmias with concomitant digoxin use. ECG changes may include a spectrum of ventricular arrhythmias (extrasystoles, tachycardia) and atrial arrhythmias (atrial fibrillation, supraventricular tachycardia), as well as torsades de pointes. Neurologic findings may include positive Chvostek's and Trousseau's signs, tremors, myoclonic jerks, seizures, and eventually coma.

Associated electrolyte abnormalities. Clinical hypomagnesemia may coexist with a combination of electrolyte abnormalities, which may help confirm the diagnosis. Hypomagnesemia occurs in 42% of patients with **hypokalemia**. When **hypokalemia** and **hypocalcemia** accompany magnesium depletion, neither can be corrected unless the magnesium deficit is repleted first. Hypomagnesemia appears to increase renal potassium wasting. It also blunts the secretion of parathyroid hormone (PTH), as well as responsiveness to PTH's peripheral action; this explains the concurrence of hypomagnesemia and hypocalcemia.

Measuring magnesium levels. Serum magnesium should be monitored in the following groups:

- All patients in critical care units

- All patients at risk for depletion (those with diabetes or alcoholism)

- All patients receiving drugs associated with magnesium loss

Note, however, that only 1% of the body's magnesium is present in the extracellular fluid; most is contained in muscle and bone. Between 15% and 30% of the intracellular pool in skeletal muscle is exchangeable with the extracellular fluid.

Thus, since serum magnesium reflects only 1% of total body magnesium, its measurement may not adequately reflect total stores. In fact, a normal serum magnesium level does not preclude a substantial deficit — especially in a person with symptoms of magnesium deficiency.

Confirmatory tests in equivocal clinical situations include those for urinary excretion and magnesium deprivation (Figure 11-1). The detection of magnesium deficiency may be improved when urinary excretion of magnesium is measured simultaneously with serum levels of magnesium. Low magnesium levels in the urine, much like low sodium levels, indicate increased renal reabsorption of magnesium in response to depletion.

Replacement therapy. A patient with a low serum magnesium level needs replacement therapy. Oral replacement is preferable to IV or IM replacement unless there is evidence of significant cardiac or neuromuscular effects. We continue oral replacement for 3 to 4 days, regardless of serum magnesium levels, to ensure that body stores are completely replenished.

Table 11-3 shows three possible regimens for magnesium replacement. Since serum magnesium levels rely on renal excretion, exercise caution when using replacement regimens in any patient with decreased renal function.

CASE 11-1. Hypomagnesemia Secondary to Alcohol Abuse, Diarrhea, and Chronic Pancreatitis

A 34-year-old man with a 10-year history of alcohol abuse presents after 2 weeks of binge drinking. He has had no alcohol for the past 5 days and is experiencing loss of appetite, weakness, and progressive agitation. Although he has a history of chronic pancreatitis, he has stopped taking pancreatic enzyme supplementation. Diarrhea with possible malabsorption has recently developed.

Physical examination. Sinus tachycardia is present. His abdomen is tender to palpation in the epigastrium; bowel sounds are normal without guarding. The stool examination is guaiac-negative. He is agitated with a symmetric increase in deep tendon reflexes and is also confused without any focal neurologic findings. Although Chvostek's and Trousseau's signs are positive, the rest of the examination is unremarkable.

Laboratory findings. Glucose, 250 mg/dL; sodium, 136 mmol/L; potassium, 2.8 mmol/L; chloride, 101 mmol/L; magnesium, 1 mEq/L; total calcium, 7.6 mg/dL; serum albumin, 2.7 g/dL; bicarbonate, 24 mEq/L; BUN, 7 mg/dL; creatinine, 0.7 mg/dL.

Figure 11-1. Documenting magnesium depletion when the serum magnesium level is equivocal

A normal serum magnesium level despite a clinical situation suggesting magnesium depletion is not uncommon. Measurement of magnesium and creatinine (the creatinine is to ensure complete collection) in the urine over 12 to 24 hours may assist with the diagnosis of hypomagnesemia. Magnesium depletion is reminiscent of potassium depletion, since potassium and magnesium are distributed primarily as intracellular ions. Thus, if you suspect magnesium depletion and serum magnesium levels are equivocal (as in an alcoholic patient or a patient taking diuretics), the following algorithm should be pursued. If you are in doubt, careful magnesium repletion is the best course with a repeat of serum and urine studies during and after treatment.

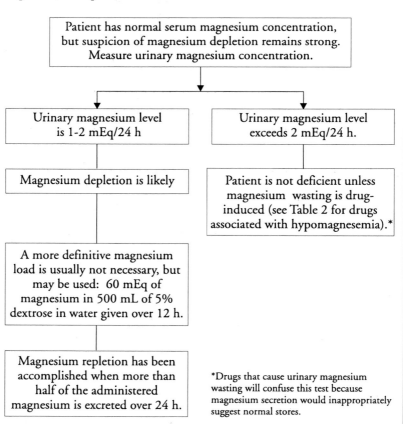

Patient has normal serum magnesium concentration, but suspicion of magnesium depletion remains strong. Measure urinary magnesium concentration.

Urinary magnesium level is 1-2 mEq/24 h

Urinary magnesium level exceeds 2 mEq/24 h.

Magnesium depletion is likely

Patient is not deficient unless magnesium wasting is drug-induced (see Table 2 for drugs associated with hypomagnesemia).*

A more definitive magnesium load is usually not necessary, but may be used: 60 mEq of magnesium in 500 mL of 5% dextrose in water given over 12 h.

Magnesium repletion has been accomplished when more than half of the administered magnesium is excreted over 24 h.

*Drugs that cause urinary magnesium wasting will confuse this test because magnesium secretion would inappropriately suggest normal stores.

The patient's serum amylase and lipase levels are normal. In addition, the aspartate aminotransferase and alanine aminotransferase levels are minimally elevated.

Diagnosis. The clinical situation in concert with the various electrolyte abnormalities is very helpful in reaching a specific diagnosis. This patient has a number of features responsible for magnesium depletion, including:

- Both acute and chronic alcohol abuse complicated by alcohol withdrawal

- Poor dietary intake

- Diarrhea

- Possible recurrent malabsorption from chronic pancreatitis

- Simultaneous hypomagnesemia, hypokalemia, and hypocalcemia

Therapy. This patient is manifesting serious end-organ dysfunction secondary to magnesium depletion — neuromuscular irritability from the hypomagnesemia and hypocalcemia with hyperactive reflexes and positive Chvostek's and Trousseau's signs. The decision to replace the magnesium orally or parenterally is based on the clinical manifestations that indicate the severity of hypomagnesemia, rather than on the

Table 11-3. Replacement therapy for hypomagnesemic patients

Route/approach	Regimen
Oral/dietary	Magnesium oxide, 400-mg tablet containing approximately 20 mEq of elemental magnesium, 4 to 6 times daily; magnesium sulfate and gluconate may cause less diarrhea
Intravenous	Magnesium sulfate, 2 g (22 mg or 4 mL of 50% magnesium sulfate in a 100 mL solution) IV over 10 minutes, followed by a continuous infusion over the next 6 h of 5 g diluted in saline or in 5% dextrose in water
Flink regimen	Loading dose: 6 g (22 mmol) of magnesium sulfate in 1,000 mL of 5% dextrose in water over 3 h, followed by 10 g (40 mmol) of magnesium sulfate in 2,000 mL of 5% dextrose in water over 24 hours; then, 6 g of magnesium sulfate diluted from a 10% or 20% solution over 24 h daily for the next 3 days

absolute serum levels. Also, it is likely that the **hypokalemia** and **hypocalcemia** will be refractory to treatment unless the magnesium is repleted. Therefore, in this case, more vigorous parenteral replacement of magnesium is warranted.

Replacement regimen. Magnesium sulfate ($MgSO_4.7H_2O$), the standard preparation for repletion, is available in solutions ranging from 10% to 50% concentrations. The former contains 1 g of $MgSO_4.7H_2O$, which is equivalent to 98.66 mg of elemental magnesium, 8.1 mEq of magnesium, or 4 mmol of magnesium.

Magnesium may be administered intramuscularly, but the injections are quite painful. A commonly used regimen for IV magnesium replacement was proposed by Flink. As a loading dose, 6 g of magnesium sulfate (12 mL of the 50% solution of $MgSO_4.7H_2O$) in 1,000 mL of 5% dextrose in water is given IV over 3 hours. This is followed by 10 g (20 mL of the 50% solution) in 2,000 mL of 5% dextrose in water over the next 24 hours.

Subsequently, 6 g of magnesium sulfate diluted from a 10% or 20% solution over 24 hours is given daily for the next 3 days. Should tetany or seizures develop, magnesium may be replaced at a more rapid rate.

Magnesium replacement therapy may be complicated by hypotension and hypermagnesemia. Therefore, it is important to monitor serum magnesium levels serially, as well as the vital signs, ECG, and deep tendon reflexes. Any deficit in **renal function** may lead to hypermagnesemia, in which case a reduction in the replacement dosage is warranted.

CASE 11-2. Hypomagnesemia following an MI in a Hyperglycemic Man Taking Digoxin and Diuretics

A 56-year-old, moderately obese man with non-insulin-dependent diabetes comes to the emergency department with acute onset of severe, crushing substernal chest pain. The ECG is consistent with an acute anterior wall myocardial infarction (MI). The patient has been taking hydrochlorothiazide (25 mg/d), a calcium channel blocker for hypertension, and digoxin (0.25 mg/d) for about 5 years. He takes only an oral hypoglycemic agent, although his glycosylated hemoglobin value exceeds 10% and he has refused insulin therapy. He takes no other medications.

Physical examination. Blood pressure, 158/104 mm Hg; pulse, 96 beats per minute and regular; respiratory rate, 18 breaths per minute; temperature, 37° C (98.6° F). The patient has mild diabetic retinopathy, but the rest of the head and neck examination is unremarkable. There are a few scattered basilar rales in the lungs.

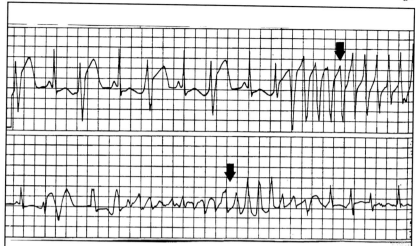

Figure 11-2. These rhythm strips are classic for torsades de pointes (arrows). Note that the axes of the QRS complexes appear to rotate around a central point. Although there are many causes of torsades de pointes, magnesium depletion may be the sole culprit in any given patient.

Cardiac evaluation reveals left ventricular hypertrophy on palpation, with an S_4, and an apical grade 2/6 systolic murmur transmitted to the axilla. Results of the abdominal and peripheral examination are normal except for mild symmetric diabetic neuropathy.

This patient was about to be taken to the cast lab when an abnormal rhythm was discovered on the ECG (Figure 11-2).

Laboratory findings. Sodium, 138 mmol/L; potassium, 3.1 mmol/L; chloride, 106 mmol/L; bicarbonate, 102 mEq/L; glucose, 300 mg/dL; BUN, 18 mg/dL; creatinine, 1.6 mg/dL. Serum calcium level is normal; the magnesium level is 1 mEq/L.

Diagnosis. Magnesium deficiency makes patients especially prone to digoxin-related arrhythmias, and this sensitivity is heightened by ischemia. This patient has a number of reasons to be magnesium deficient. He is taking diuretics and digoxin, and he is under an osmotic diuresis from the chronic hyperglycemia.

Therapy. Life-threatening arrhythmias in the setting of hypomagnesemia constitute a medical emergency requiring immediate intervention. IV magnesium sulfate may be administered as 20 mL of a 20% solution or 2 g over 1 to 2 minutes. This is followed by an infusion of 5 to 10 g over the next 6 to 12 hours with cautious monitoring.

An alternative method of rapid IV magnesium loading, especially useful when seizures are secondary to hypomagnesemia, is a slow IV bolus of 4 mL of a 50% solution of magnesium sulfate (2 g) over 10 minutes followed by a continuous infusion as above. Saline solution may be used as a diluent whenever excess IV glucose should be avoided, as in this case.

In patients with impaired renal function, monitoring is imperative to prevent overcorrection of the hypomagnesemia — especially when parenteral replacement is vigorous.

CASE 11-3. Hypomagnesemia in Patient with AIDS Taking Foscarnet

A 32-year-old man with AIDS and a CD4 count of 75/mL presents with progressive weakness over the last month. The clinical course has been complicated by AIDS-associated diarrhea of unknown cause and by cytomegalovirus (CMV) retinitis, for which he is receiving foscarnet therapy. He has been so ill recently that his dietary intake has declined, and he has discontinued the foscarnet.

Physical examination. The patient is afebrile, and his vital signs are otherwise normal. The head and neck examination is unremarkable, and his lungs are clear to percussion and auscultation. Cardiac and abdominal examinations are normal; neurologic examination shows brisk but symmetric deep tendon reflexes. There is a generalized decrease in muscle strength to 3/5 in all muscle groups tested.

Laboratory findings. Sodium, 130 mmol/L; potassium, 2.9 mmol/L; chloride, 106 mmol/L; bicarbonate, 18 mEq/L; glucose, 80 mg/dL; BUN, 30 mg/dL; creatinine 1.4 mg/dL. His serum magnesium level is 1.2 mEq/L.

Since magnesium deficiency was expected, the amounts of magnesium and creatinine in the urine over 24 hours were determined. Urinary magnesium level was 2 mEq/24 h specimen; this suggested magnesium depletion, especially with foscarnet treatment.

Diagnosis. Magnesium depletion can result from either GI or renal causes, and the amount of magnesium in the urine over 24 hours is quite helpful in making this distinction. A low serum magnesium level that is accompanied by small amounts of magnesium collected in the urine over 24 hours signifies a GI cause of magnesium loss with a normal renal response. Conversely, large amounts of magnesium collected in the urine over 24 hours with hypomagnesemia indicate renal wasting of magnesium from any of several disease states or drugs.

The factors contributing to hypomagnesemia in persons with AIDS are:

- Chronic diarrhea

- Malnutrition

- Steatorrhea

Foscarnet, a commonly used antiviral agent against CMV, has also been implicated in the pathogenesis of hypomagnesemia; the incidence of this complication is at least 15%. Although the exact mechanism is unknown, the chelation of magnesium ions may be involved. Foscarnet is nephrotoxic, so its use could result in hypomagnesemia from renal magnesium wasting. Since this patient discontinued taking foscarnet, the loss from the urine may have stopped before the urine collection.

Therapy. Treatment should include long-term magnesium replacement therapy. An oral agent, such as magnesium oxide (containing roughly 20 mEq of elemental magnesium) given as 400-mg tablet four to six times a day, is the preferred mode. However, it could potentially worsen the diarrhea, necessitating one of the parenteral regimens described in Table 11-3.

Hypermagnesemia

While hypomagnesemia is fairly common, hypermagnesemia may be the most rare of all clinical electrolyte abnormalities. Hypermagnesemia develops most often in patients with increased magnesium intake coupled with a decreased renal excretion. It may occur, for example, in a patient on dialysis taking magnesium-containing laxatives to combat constipation. Hypermagnesemia secondary to magnesium sulfate therapy for preeclampsia has been reported occasionally. Other settings in which hypermagnesemia can develop include:

- A severe catabolic state, such as rhabdomyolysis

- Decreased magnesium excretion in acute or chronic renal failure

Clinical manifestations. Symptoms vary; a patient may be asymptomatic or in coma or cardiac arrest. One important clinical pearl to keep in mind: if the hypermagnesemic patient is hypotensive, in coma, or in shock, he or she will not have deep tendon reflexes. If reflexes are present, consider a cause other than excess magnesium for the vascular or CNS abnormality.

Treatment. Therapy is straightforward. In asymptomatic patients with elevated magnesium levels, remove exogenous sources of magnesium and search for the underlying cause. When more serious complications arise, treat as you would for hyperkalemia. For example, give IV calcium as a gluconate or chloride salt if ECG abnormalities are present (peaked T waves, loss of P waves, or widened QRS complexes); give parenteral insulin-glucose to shift magnesium into cells; and provide dialysis for patients who have severe hypermagnesemia after stabilization of the ECG findings.

Case 11-4. Hypermagnesemia in a Patient on Hemodialysis

The patient is a 67-year-old woman on hemodialysis admitted for congestive heart failure (CHF) and constipation. Her past medical history includes renal failure from vascular disease, CAD with an ejection fraction of 30%, and recurrent CHF. She has had occasional hypotension while receiving dialysis, but no other problems have been noted. She has been taking captopril (25 mg twice a day) for her heart failure and a multivitamin.

Physical examination. The patient was not in acute distress. Her blood pressure was 140/92 mm Hg, pulse was 98 beats per minute and regular, and respiratory rate was 24 breaths per minute. There was some elevation of her jugular venous pulse at 30 degrees, scattered bibasilar rales, cardiomegaly, an S_3 gallop and a grade 2/6 mitral regurgitation murmur.

Laboratory findings. Despite erythropoietin, her hematocrit value had decreased to 30%. Levels of serum electrolytes, albumin, and calcium were normal; BUN was 60 mg/dL, creatinine, 4.7 mg/dL. On rectal examination, the patient had impacted stool, but she did not respond to a soapsuds enema. She had received a number of magnesium-containing enemas, and her daughter reported that her intake at home included magnesium-containing antacids and laxatives.

Complications. A few hours after admission, the patient began to vomit and have some diarrhea; she became hypotensive and experienced chest pain. Deep tendon reflexes were absent. An acute MI was suspected. Her serum magnesium level was 9 mEq/L.

Diagnosis. This patient with severely impaired renal function was taking long-term magnesium-containing compounds and was also given magnesium by enema. The vomiting, hypotension, and absence of deep tendon reflexes should have alerted the physicians to the possibility of hypermagnesemia. A high index of suspicion coupled with prompt monitoring of magnesium level and ECG is essential.

Therapy. Once diagnosed, hypermagnesemia is treated in the same way as hyperkalemia. IV calcium gluconate, insulin, and dextrose are immediately administered. Saline and furosemide increase magnesium excretion, and hemodialysis can effectively remove magnesium — especially if there is concurrent renal insufficiency.

This patient's renal failure and dependence on dialysis led to emergent dialysis against a low magnesium bath. The patient and her family were cautioned against the use of magnesium-containing antacids and laxatives.

Suggested Reading

1. Agus ZS. Hypomagnesemia. *J Am Soc Nephrol.* 1999; 10:1616-1622.

2. Agus ZS, Kelepouris E, Dukes I, et al. Cytosolic magnesium modulates calcium channel activity in mammalian ventricular cells. *Am J Physiol.* 1989; 256:C452-C455.

3. Al-Ghamdi SMG, Cameron ECC, Sutton RAL. Magnesium deficiency: pathophysiologic and clinical overview. *Am J Kidney Dis.* 1994: 24: 737-752.

4. Bohmer T, Mathiesen B. Magnesium deficiency in chronic alcoholic patients uncovered by an intravenous loading test. *Scand J Clin Lab Invest.* 1982; 42: 633-636.

5. DeMarchi S, Cecchin E, Basile A, et al. Renal tubular dysfunction in chronic alcohol abuse: effect of abstinence. *N Engl J Med.* 1993; 329: 1927-1934.

6. England MR, Gordon G, Salem M, Chernow B. Magnesium administration and dysrhythmias after cardiac surgery. *JAMA.* 1992; 268: 2395-2402.

7. Fink BE. Magnesium deficiency. Etiology and clinical spectrum. *Acta Med Scand.* 1981: 647 (suppl): 125-137.

8. Gearhart MO, Song TB. Foscarnet-induced severe hypomagnesemia and other electrolyte disorders. *Ann Pharmacother.* 1993; 27: 285-289.

9. Hebert P, Mehta N, Wang J. Functional magnesium deficiency in critically ill patients identified using a magnesium-loading test. *Crit Care Med.* 1997; 25:749-755.

10. Nadler JL, Rude RK. Disorders of magnesium metabolism. *Endocrinol Metab Clin North Am.* 1995;24:623-641.

11. Ryzen E, Elkayam U, Rude RK. Low blood mononuclear cell magnesium in intensive cardiac care unit patients. *Am Heart J.* 1986; 111: 475-480.

12. Rutecki GW, Whittier FC. Hyperkalemia: how to identify and correct the underlying cause. *Consultant* 1996; 36: 564-573.

13. Whang R, Oei TO, Aikawa JK, et al. Predictors of clinical hypomagnesemia, hypokalemia, hypophosphatemia, hyponatremia, and hypocalcemia. *Arch Intern Med.* 1984; 144: 1794-1796.

14. Whang R, Ryder KW. Frequency of hypomagnesemia and hypermagnesemia: requested vs. routine. *JAMA.* 1990; 263: 3063-3064.

15. Wong ET, Rude RK, Singer FR, et al. A high prevalence of hypomagnesemia in hospitalized patients. *Am J Clin Pathol.* 1983; 79: 348-352.

16. Woods KL, Fletcher S, Roffe C, et al. Intravenous magnesium sulfate in suspected myocardial infarction: results of the second Leicester Intravenous Magnesium Intervention Trial (LIMIT-2). *Lancet.* 1992; 339:1553-1558.

12. The Rules of Three in Oliguria
How to Use This Technique for Evaluation

How to use this technique for evaluation

Oliguria is defined as a decrease in urine flow to less than 400 mL/d ($\pm$ 100 mL) or less than 20 mL/hr. This condition occurs in such a wide variety of clinical settings and with so many associated diseases that it is essential to take a systematic approach to possible causes.

For an understandable and systematic evaluation of oliguria, we present the Rules of Three: three categories of oliguria; three basic, noninvasive tools used for evaluation and differentiation; and three practical clinical maxims (Table 12-1). We will then apply these Rules of Three to specific case studies to increase their utility in clinical situations.

The Rules of Three have additional clinical advantages. First, the diagnostic procedures have supplanted the intravenous pyelogram or contrast CT as imaging studies for evaluating oliguria, thus obviating the possibility of adverse reactions to contrast. Second, these procedures are inexpensive and devoid of complications. Finally, their use can be expanded, with reliable diagnostic accuracy, to the evaluation of elevated levels of blood urea nitrogen and serum creatinine (azotemia) or of proteinuria. These advantages make the Rules of Three a necessary part of the primary physician's repertoire.

The three categories of oliguria

A decrease in urinary output results from one of three general causes: postrenal, prerenal, or renal (renal parenchymal insufficiency) — or a combination thereof. The order in which you evaluate these three causes is critical.

Postrenal failure, or obstruction to urinary flow, can occur at any level of the urinary tract. The term postrenal is used because the decrease in urinary flow occurs after urine has been produced by the kidney. Many common conditions, such as *prostatic hypertrophy* or *urinary obstruction* caused by stones or tumor, may present as postrenal disease with oliguria (Table 12-2).

Table 12-1. The Rules of Three

Three Categories of Oliguria
- Postrenal
- Prerenal
- Renal (parenchymal insufficiency)

Three Noninvasive Diagnostic Tools
- History and physical examination
- Ultrasonography
- Urinalysis with urinary electrolytes

Three Clinical Maxims
- All oliguria is considered obstructive until proved otherwise.
- Only after postrenal and prerenal causes are eliminated can one pursue the third category: renal parenchymal insufficiency.
- A carefully done urinalysis, using a fresh specimen, is critical in the workup of every oliguric patient.

Rule out postrenal causes of oliguria by considering the **first clinical maxim: all oliguria is considered to be obstructive until proved otherwise.** This point is particularly important, since early diagnosis and prompt correction of obstructive causes will result in minimal permanent kidney damage. Unfortunately, the converse applies: uncorrected obstruction can lead to irreversible renal failure.

Prerenal failure. In prerenal failure, oliguria is due to an abnormality that affects the perfusion of normal renal parenchyma (Table 12-3). The condition may be corrected with restoration of volume and circulatory deficits. **Volume contraction** from nausea (sufficient to restrict fluid intake), vomiting, use of diuretics, or blood loss leads to a number of pathophysiologic responses that are characteristic of prerenal states. These include intrarenal vasoconstriction with a subsequent decrease in renal blood flow.

Further, a **decrease in cardiac output** may result in decreased glomerular filtration and the increased production of renal-active hormones (e.g., angiotensin II, antidiuretic hormone, and aldosterone), all of which decrease urinary volume. The prerenal responses all become normalized with correction of the circulatory insufficiency.

The same sequence of events commonly occurs in *volume-expanded states,* such as congestive heart failure, cirrhosis, and nephrotic syndrome. Despite the excess of total body volume in these conditions, the common denominator is **ineffective circulating arterial volume,** which leads to the same renal dynamics as does volume contraction. Correction of the cardiac, hepatic, or renal problem reverses the prerenal state, since the result of all these diverse conditions is a decrease in urine output with **normally** functioning renal parenchyma.

One hallmark of prerenal oliguria is that the BUN to creatinine ratio usually exceeds the normal of 10:1; frequently, it is 15:1, 20:1, or greater.

Therefore, a BUN level of 40 mg/dL and a simultaneous serum creatinine value of 2 mg/dL is a socalled a prerenal ratio (20:1).

Renal parenchymal insufficiency. Reversible oliguria will never be overlooked if you adhere to the **second clinical maxim: only after post-renal and prerenal causes are eliminated can one pursue the third general category of oliguria—renal parenchymal insufficiency.** Intra-renal failure encompasses a wide spectrum of diseases, as well as a wide spectrum of treatments (Table 12-4). For ease of classification, the renal parenchymal category of oliguria can be subdivided into two major groups: tubulointerstitial disease and glomerular disease. Both may be either acute or chronic.

The three noninvasive tools

In order to differentiate the features of these three renal categories, you must have knowledge of the three basic noninvasive tools used for evaluation of oliguria: history and physical examination, ultrasonography of the kidneys, and urinalysis with spot urine electrolytes.

History and physical examination. A history of volume contraction (use of diuretics, protracted nausea and/or vomiting, decreased oral intake, Addison's disease) can indicate prerenal causes. Difficulty with the initiation of urinary stream, dribbling, a history of solitary kidney or renal lithiasis can lead to the diagnosis of postrenal insufficiency.

Table 12-2. Postrenal causes of oliguria

Lower urinary tract:

Urethral disease (stricture or valve disorder)

Prostate (benign or malignant enlargement)

Bladder (neurogenic dysfunction, malignancy, or effect of parasympatholytic drugs)

Upper urinary tract:

Extrinsic obstruction of collecting system

Malignant disease (metastatic, lymphoma, ovarian, uterine, urethral)

Inflammatory (tuberculosis, sarcoidosis, abscess)

Anatomic (aberrant vessels, pregnancy)

Other (retroperitoneal fibrosis, radiation)

Intrinsic obstruction of collecting system

Stones

Blood clots

Papillae

Fungus balls

Intraluminal tumor

If postrenal and prerenal causes are not evident from the history, the specific type of renal parenchymal disease may become apparent following appropriate questions and associations. For example, a thorough **drug history** is essential, since many patients with renal failure have a clear-cut exposure to a nephrotoxic medication (eg, a nonsteroidal anti-inflammatory drug).

The association of renal parenchymal injury with a history of systemic disease is also valuable. **Diabetes mellitus** is the most common cause of chronic glomerular injury in this country. Among persons undergoing long-term dialysis, 25% to 33% have renal injury associated with diabetes of 10 years' standing or longer. The history and clinical presentation of these patients are usually so classic that a noninvasive workup alone is virtually diagnostic.

Table 12-3. Prerenal causes of oliguria
Decreased vascular volume
Blood loss
Volume loss (eg, use of diuretics, vomiting, Addison's disease)
Third space loss of fluid (eg, from pancreatitis, postoperative, burns)
Increased vascular volume with ineffective circulation
Cardiac (congestive heart failure)
Nephrotic syndrome
Cirrhosis
Drugs
NSAIDs
Angiotensin converting enzyme inhibitors
Others, (eg, tetracycline, prednisone)

The physical exam may provide clues to many diverse diseases that will categorize the oliguria in one of the three basic groups. **A postural decrease in blood pressure** is one of the most important findings and may uncover subtle volume depletion. Compare the supine BP and pulse with the seated or standing values; look for a 10-mm Hg drop in systolic pressure and/or an increase of 10 beats per minute in the pulse on the assumption of upright posture. This aspect of the physical exam may be the most important determinant for uncovering a prerenal cause for oliguria. Look also for a **rash** from drug-induced interstitial nephritis or for skin changes in the lower extremity (eg, livedo reticularis); the latter may be found with cholesterol embolization.

Ultrasonography. One of the most attractive features of ultrasonography is its freedom from complications—unlike its imaging predecessor, the intravenous pyelogram. This feature, along with affordability and availability, makes ultrasonography the gold standard for renal imaging in oliguria. It is extremely sensitive and specific in ruling out postrenal causes of oliguria and, therefore, has become the initial test of choice for the diagnosis of obstruction. A CT scan may accomplish the same goals, but should be done without contrast.

Additional information provided by this modality includes the differentiation between acute and chronic renal disease, based on kidney size. Small kidneys, as visualized by ultrasound, are a tip-off to the fact that oliguria is chronic and, therefore, less reversible. Increased renal echogenicity on ultrasonographic examination (intensified kidney echoes that are as dense as liver echoes) signifies renal parenchymal disease.

By showing a disparity in size between kidneys (2 cm or greater), ultrasonography may uncover occult renovascular disease. This is represented by loss of mass in the smaller kidney, the result of ischemic injury. Ultrasonography also identifies the patient with a solitary kidney who might develop oliguria or even anuria during the passage of a stone or clot.

Again, a computed tomographic scan (CT) may be used to obtain the same information. It may even provide better imaging in some circumstances. However, it is more expensive and carries risk if intravenous contrast is given.

Urinalysis. The third noninvasive test consists of evaluating a few

---

Table 12-4. Renal causes of oliguria

Acute

  Tubulointerstitial

    Acute tubular necrosis (eg, rhabdomyolysis, shock)

    Interstitial nephritis (from drugs, infection)

    Nephrotoxins (ethylene glycol, contrast media)

    Pregnancy-associated (hemorrhage)

    Other (cholesterol emboli)

  Glomerular

    Primary glomerular diseases (eg, following streptococcal infection; membranoproliferative glomerulonephritis)

Chronic

  Tubulointerstitial

    Nephrosclerosis, vascular disease (ischemic nephropathy)

    Interstitial nephritis (eg, from analgesics)

    Toxins

  Glomerular

    Any chronic glomerular disease (eg, focal glomerulosclerosis, membranoproliferative glomerulonephritis, diabetes mellitus)

milliliters of urine before any therapy is undertaken. In fact, this procedure leads to the **third clinical maxim: a carefully done urinalysis,
using a fresh specimen, is critical in the workup of every
oliguric patient.** This test is particularly helpful in categorizing renal
parenchymal disease (glomerular or tubulointerstitial) after you have
eliminated postrenal and prerenal causes. A dipstick reaction for urinary
protein of 3+ to 4+ and the presence of red blood cell casts in the urine
are pathognomonic of oliguria secondary to a glomerular disorder. You
can further corroborate this diagnosis by testing a 24-hour urine collection for protein; the dipstick value suggests that it will contain 2 g or
more, which is consistent with glomerular disease. This finding identifies
a damaged glomerulus as the leakage site of large amounts of protein
and RBC casts into the urine.

A low grade of proteinuria seen on the dipstick (eg, 1+ to 2+, which
is equivalent to less than 1.5 g of protein in a 24-hour specimen) is
suggestive of renal parenchymal disease localized to the interstitium and
tubules, rather than the glomerulus. Low-grade dip-stick proteinuria
coupled with coarsely granular casts and renal tubular epithelial cells
from injured tubules can be diagnostic of acute tubular necrosis (ATN),
which is a common cause of renal oliguria in hospitalized patients.

Low-grade proteinuria associated with eosinophils in the plasma or
urine may be diagnostic of acute interstitial nephritis from drugs. Completely normal results of urinalysis constitute strong evidence that the
oliguria is potentially reversible and not due to renal parenchymal
disease.

A few milliliters of urine can also provide valuable information when
sent for a spot test for electrolytes (eg, sodium, creatinine, and osmolality). The fractional excretion of sodium (FENa), which helps to distinguish between renal and prerenal failure, is determined by dividing the
urinary to plasma sodium ratio by the urinary to plasma creatinine ratio
and multiplying by 100. In acute and chronic renal failure, the FENa
would be high (greater than 2); in prerenal failure, it would be 1 or less.

The renal failure index is a slight variation on the same theme. It is
derived by dividing the urinary creatinine concentration by that of the
serum creatinine and then dividing the urinary sodium by the resulting
quotient. The renal failure index is essentially equivalent to the FENa,
and a given institution may arbitrarily choose to use one or the other.

As an example, a normal kidney affected by decreased arterial
volume (prerenal failure) will vigorously resorb sodium and thereby
decrease urinary sodium values to less than 10 mEq/L; the FENa would
be less than 1. The osmolality of this prerenal urine would be 500
mOsm/kg water or greater.

Conversely, if a kidney has sustained an injury resulting in myoglobinuric renal failure, or ATN, the tubules will be rendered ineffective for the reabsorption of sodium and concentration of urine. In fact, this disease is an excellent example of one that utilizes the three diagnostic tools for oliguria: Findings from history (muscle injury) and physical exam (no postural drop in BP, evidence of muscle injury); ultrasonography (no obstruction, kidneys of normal size with renal disease); measurement of urinary electrolytes (an increase in urinary sodium, FENa value, or renal failure index); and urinalysis results (protein in urine, 1+ to 2+ by dipstick; and coarse, granular, pigmented casts) are pathognomonic for parenchymal renal disease secondary to myoglobin, obviating the need for invasive workup.

We will now apply the Rules of Three to five common clinical situations.

Case 12-1. A 65-year-old Man with Hypertension and Prostatic Obstruction

A man, aged 65, was being followed for essential hypertension. His chief complaint was a decrease in urination during the 6 months since he was last seen. This decrease had recently worsened and was now associated with decreased appetite and weight gain due to edema. On being questioned, the patient admitted that he had had nocturia, urinary frequency, a significantly decreased strength of urinary stream, and occasional dribbling during this 6-month period. The only medication he had been taking was hydrochlorothiazide, 25 mg/d, which kept his hypertension in good control. There was no other significant medical history.

Examination revealed supine BP, 160/102 mm Hg and pulse, 80 beats per minute; standing BP, 164/104 mm Hg and pulse, 80 beats per minute; grade I hypertensive retinopathy; mild left ventricular hypertrophy on palpation, sustained left ventricular impulse with S_4; peripheral ankle edema 1+ to 2+; and a lower abdominal mass on palpation and percussion. At the patient's last visit, BUN and serum creatinine levels had been 19 mg/dL and 1.6 mg/dL, respectively; they were now 44 mg/dL and 3.8 mg/dL. Prostate specific antigen (PSA) was normal.

The first maxim, all oliguria is considered obstructive until proved otherwise, led to ultrasonography. This showed a 10.8-cm right kidney, a 10.7-cm left kidney, and bilateral hydronephrosis. On urinalysis, dipstick reaction for protein was 1+; microscopic examination revealed 5 to 10 WBCs per high-power field and 5 to 10 RBCs; occasional finely granular casts were noted, but no coarse casts. The bladder was obstructed, and placement of a Foley catheter resulted in production of more than 4 liters of urine in 24 hours.

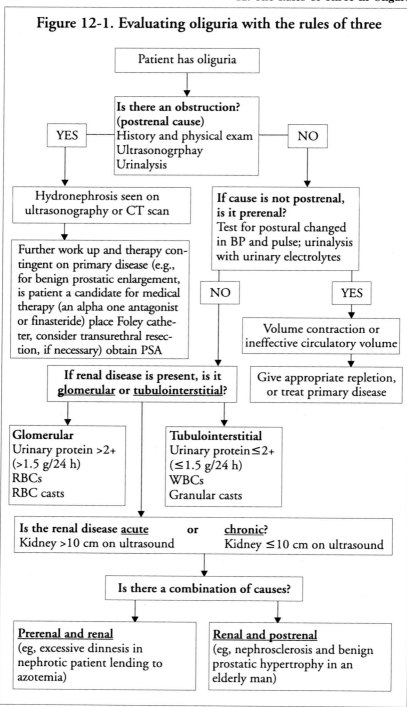

Figure 12-1. Evaluating oliguria with the rules of three

Patient has oliguria

Is there an obstruction?
(postrenal cause)
History and physical exam
Ultrasonogrphay
Urinalysis

YES — NO

Hydronephrosis seen on ultrasonography or CT scan

If cause is not postrenal, is it prerenal?
Test for postural changed in BP and pulse; urinalysis with urinary electrolytes

Further work up and therapy contingent on primary disease (e.g., for benign prostatic enlargement, is patient a candidate for medical therapy (an alpha one antagonist or finasteride) place Foley catheter, consider transurethral resection, if necessary) obtain PSA

NO   YES

Volume contraction or ineffective circulatory volume

If renal disease is present, is it glomerular or tubulointerstitial?

Give appropriate repletion, or treat primary disease

Glomerular
Urinary protein >2+
(>1.5 g/24 h)
RBCs
RBC casts

Tubulointerstitial
Urinary protein ≤2+
(≤1.5 g/24 h)
WBCs
Granular casts

Is the renal disease acute   or   chronic?
Kidney >10 cm on ultrasound   Kidney ≤10 cm on ultrasound

Is there a combination of causes?

Prerenal and renal
(eg, excessive dinness in nephrotic patient lending to azotemia)

Renal and postrenal
(eg, nephrosclerosis and benign prostatic hypertrophy in an elderly man)

After 48 hours, the BUN and serum creatinine returned to baseline values (17 mg/dL and 1.5 mg/dL, respectively). Transurethral resection corrected the obstruction.

Discussion. This is a typical presentation of prostatic obstruction, a problem that brings many men to primary care physicians. This case also demonstrates that relief of a postrenal disorder may completely restore normal renal function. Milder symptoms of obstruction or prostatic hypertrophy may be treated medically with alpha-1-blockers or finasteride.

Two additional points concerning postrenal failure are extremely important: first, patients may be completely asymptomatic. Elevated BUN or serum creatinine values or suggestive mild complaints may be caused by the obstruction. Second, patients with high-grade obstruction may continue to excrete significant amounts of urine. It is a common misconception that obstruction is always associated with oliguria. Therefore, consider obstruction when any renal abnormality is present, regardless of presenting symptoms and signs.

Case 12-2. A 72-year-old Woman with CHF and Nonobstructive Oliguria

A woman, aged 72, who resides in an extended care facility had a recent history of lethargy and decreased oral intake. She recovered from a stroke a year ago and was rehabilitated, with minimal residual dysfunction. Because of a history of mild congestive heart failure, she took maintenance dosages of furosemide (40 mg/d) and digoxin (0.125 mg daily). During the past week, she had complained of an upset stomach and had been vomiting for 2 to 3 days. Her urine output had decreased dramatically over the past week.

The patient's supine BP was 150/80 mm Hg and pulse 98 beats per minute; seated BP was 135/76 mm Hg and pulse 118 beats per minute. She complained of dizziness while sitting and preferred to lie supine. She was somewhat lethargic but arousable and oriented. Slight right-sided weakness remained from a previous stroke, but there were no new focal neurologic signs. Her lungs were clear, and her jugular pulse was flat at 30 degrees of elevation. Results of her cardiac examination were normal. There was no peripheral edema, but her medical records documented edema (2+) in the past.

Even though findings from this patient's history and physical exam did not suggest an obstruction, an appropriate workup demands ruling out a postrenal cause of oliguria. Renal ultrasonographic examination showed bilateral 10-cm kidneys without hydronephrosis. At this point, a postrenal cause was eliminated.

According to the second maxim, it was then necessary to assume that the oliguria was of prerenal origin until proved otherwise. Actually, the history of decreased intake and vomiting, coupled with a postural decline in BP and tachycardia, is suggestive of a pre-renal cause. Initial laboratory tests revealed BUN, 86 mg/dL; and serum creatinine, 2 mg/dL (a ratio of 43:1). An earlier reading showed values of 24 mg/dL and 1.7 mg/dL, respectively. Electrolyte levels included sodium, 132 mEq/L; potassium, 3.4 mEq/L; bicarbonate, 32 mEq/L; and chloride, 92 mEq/L.

Urinalysis showed dipstick reaction for protein, 1+; sediment was without casts or tubular epithelial cells, evidence that tubular injury was absent. Spot test of urine showed a sodium content of 4 mEq/L and urine osmolality of 600 mOsm/kg of water. These findings were consistent with volume contraction and intact renal ability to reabsorb sodium and concentrate the urine — indicative of a prerenal condition.

Treatment. The patient was given normal saline IV, initially at 200 mL/h, and followed up serially with BP, heart and lung exams, and BUN and creatinine values. She was found to have a small duodenal ulcer and gastroesophageal reflux disease, which were treated with an H_2 blocker. The IV treatment was tapered and stopped when she was able to resume oral intake. Because of her age, care was taken not to volume overload her. The patient's BUN and creatinine values returned to baseline, her urinary sodium levels increased, and the postural decline in BP was resolved. With continued H_2 blocker therapy, the patient was able to return to her previous level of activity. She was *H. pylori* negative.

Discussion. In an office setting, the history often enables you to make a straightforward diagnosis of prerenal failure. When you are dealing with an inpatient, however, oliguria from prerenal causes (particularly postoperative) is more difficult to diagnose and manage. Even though ultrasonography effectively rules out obstruction following surgery, many clinicians forget the second maxim and assume the presence of renal parenchymal oliguria, or ATN. Thus, many patients with prerenal failure are inappropriately given diuretics or mannitol, which results in further volume contraction.

Again, urinalysis is critical, since the absence of casts makes renal parenchymal failure less likely. In hospitalized patients, nonobstructive oliguria may require consultation with a nephrologist, placement of a Swan-Ganz catheter, and/or volume loading to prevent prerenal oliguria from progressing to renal parenchymal failure. Only after a patient is treated for a prerenal state can one appropriately assess and treat renal parenchymal disease.

CASE 12-3. A 36-year-old Man with Chronic Alcoholism, Rhabdomyolysis and Myoglobinuria

A man, aged 36, with a long history of alcoholism was admitted to the hospital because of abdominal pain, nausea, and vomiting. Within 24 hours, he developed oliguria. His serum amylase and lipase values were elevated because of pancreatitis.

The patient's supine BP was 100/60 mm Hg and pulse, 120 beats per minute with a marked postural change. He was confused but without focal neurologic signs. His left lower leg was moderately swollen; it had been trapped beneath him after he became stuporous and fell, prior to admission. His upper abdomen was tender. Results of the cardiopulmonary examination were normal. After placement of a foley catheter, oliguria was noted (urine volume less than 10 mL/h).

Although the ability to insert a foley catheter often rules out prostatic obstruction, ultrasonography is still helpful. In this case, it demonstrated normal-sized kidneys (both 11.2 cm) without obstruction and with normal echogenicity. On the initial urinalysis, the dipstick demonstrated protein, 1+, and the sediment contained a few hyaline casts. Initial BUN and creatinine values were 18 mg/dL and 1.1 mg/dL, respectively. The urinary sodium level was 1 mEq/L, and osmolality was 618 mOsm/kg of water.

The patient was treated vigorously with 3 to 4 L of normal saline, IV. His urine output increased as the BUN and creatinine values became stabilized at 34 mg/dL and 2 mg/dL, respectively, within 24 hours. Two days later, he again became oliguric despite having a BP of 140/80 mm Hg without postural change. At this time, the following abnormal laboratory values were obtained: serum creatine kinase (from skeletal muscle), 15,000 U/L; and serum phosphorous, 1.6 mg/dL. There was further swelling of his left lower leg.

This patient fits into the category of renal parenchymal failure. Ultrasonography ruled out postrenal failure, and vigorous fluid repletion corrected his volume deficit. Potential prerenal causes are third spacing, nausea and vomiting, and decreased intake.

Repeated urinalysis and urinary electrolyte measurements are essential to the diagnosis. Thirty-six hours later, another urinalysis showed the same dipstick protein value in addition to numerous coarsely granular, pigmented casts and renal tubular epithelial cells that had not been seen previously. Urinary sodium increased to 60 mEq/L (FENa, 5%), and osmolality decreased to 312 mOsm/kg of water. Plasma osmolality was 316 mOsm/kg of water.

This patient had acute renal failure due to rhabdomyolysis and myoglobinuria. This diagnosis was further documented by the rise in creatine kinase (from muscle), evidence of swelling in an injured muscle group (in the left lower leg), alcoholism, and low serum phosphorus value—all risk factors for this disease. However, this diagnosis cannot be made accurately until postrenal and prerenal causes have been eliminated or managed.

Discussion. This diagnosis is important for numerous reasons. We would not want to precipitate acute renal failure by initiating diuresis in someone who is oliguric and has severe volume contraction, as was this patient on the first day. Since he had pancreatitis, third spacing could result in vasoconstriction to the kidney. In addition, once his fluids were adequately replaced, he remained oliguric, further fluid could not be given because it might lead to congestive heart failure. With a further increase of the BUN and creatinine values, the patient's oliguria and azotemia needed further treatment with dialysis. Acute parenchymal renal failure such as ATN has a significant mortality rate ($\geq 50\%$); it is reversible, but patients may require 3 to 4 weeks of medical and dialytic support.

A situation similar to ATN may occur with the use of intravenous contrast media (especially in diabetic patients with proteinunia), during postoperative hypotensive or septic states, and with the use of NSAIDs in patients with mild chronic renal disease. These conditions are diagnosed and managed in the same way.

CASE 12-4. A 42-year-old Woman Allergic to Penicillin

A woman, aged 42, complained of a rash and also noted a decrease in urine volume. She had recently been taking penicillin, which was prescribed for pharyngitis. She was otherwise healthy and had had no exposure to other medications.

The patient's BP was 146/88 mm Hg and was unchanged with posture. A generalized maculopapular rash was the only notable finding on physical exam. Screening laboratory work showed BUN and serum creatinine values of 55 mg/dL and 6 mg/dL, respectively (ratio, about 10:1).

Ultrasonography showed no obstruction; the two kidneys were each approximately 11.4 cm long, with an ultrasonagraphic pattern suggestive of renal disease. The patient had adequate oral intake, showed no postural BP changes, and did not appear to have volume contraction. Spot urinary electrolyte measurements showed a urinary sodium level of 38 mmol/L (FENa, 4%) and a urinary osmolality of 308 mOsm/kg of water (plasma osmolality, 313 mOsm/kg of water).

Urinalysis showed dipstick proteinurea (2+), finely granular casts, and on Hansel's stain, eosinophils. A CBC count with differential revealed 26% eosinophils.

Results from use of the three tools rule out either postrenal or prerenal failure. From the tests and ultrasonographic findings, the patient appeared to have acute renal parenchymal failure (of recent onset, from history and renal size) associated with a generalized rash from penicillin. This allergic state was further corroborated by the presence of eosinophils in the urine and in the plasma. In some instances, renal biopsy may be performed to demonstrate the diagnosis. This is a classic presentation of acute interstitial nephritis secondary to the use of penicillin, a renal parenchymal disorder that may be associated with systemic drug allergy.

The penicillin therapy was discontinued; the patient was admitted, and BUN/creatinine levels were followed. This disease may resolve with conservative therapy, or it may occasionally require use of corticosteroids or temporary dialysis, pending recovery. It is associated with numerous medications, including antibiotics (all of the penicillins and the blactams), NSAIDs, diuretics, anticonvulsants (phenytoin and others), captopril, allopurinol, and clofibrate.

Discussion. This case of renal oliguria demonstrates the utility of the three tools expanded by the third clinical maxim. After elimination of postrenal and prerenal causes, ultrasonography (normal renal size) and urinalysis (low-grade dipstick proteinuria) would categorize the patient's disease as acute and tubulointerstitial. Although eosinophils are found in only 10% of cases of drug-induced interstitial nephritis, it is worthwhile to search for them. Their presence is specific and diagnostic for this condition.

CASE 12-5. A 27-year-old Man with Acute Glomerular Oliguria

A hypertensive man, aged 27, came to the emergency department with oliguria (output of 320 mL/d). Lab values obtained at that time included BUN, 57 mg/dL and serum creatinine, 3.6 mg/dL. His illness appeared to have started slowly; fatigue and then decreased appetite developed over the past month, and gross hematuria had occurred 24 hours earlier.

Physical examination revealed BP supine, 180/106 mm Hg and pulse, 96 beats per minute; BP seated, 186/108 mm Hg and pulse, 97 beats per minute. Auscultation disclosed scattered rales and rhonchi and an S_4; the degree of peripheral edema was 1+.

Ultrasonography showed an 11.4-cm left kidney and an 11.1-cm right kidney, increased echogenicity, and no obstruction (denoting acute 1disease). Urinalysis revealed proteinuria (4+), 20 to 30 RBCs per high-power field, and 1 to 2 RBC casts. A 24-hour urine collection contained 3.6 g of protein.

This patient's disease fits the category of acute glomerular oliguria, which requires consultation with a nephrologist. As additional screening workup, complement values, antinuclear antibody titer, hepatitis B surface antigen titer, hepatitis C antibodies, antistreptolysin-O titer, serum protein electrophoresis and urine immuno-electrophoresis were ordered.

Even with these additional studies, a patient with this condition requires a renal biopsy for definitive diagnosis and treatment. A diagnosis of rapidly progressive glomerulonephritis (RPGN, or crescentic glomerulonephritis), for example, comprises different diseases that require different and potentially toxic therapy: patients with Wegener's granulomatosis are treated with cyclophosphamide and prednisone, whereas those with other RPGN disorders may be given boluses of corticosteroids. Glomerular diseases that are not in the RPGN group may require other types of management.

This patient's renal biopsy revealed a diagnosis of idiopathic rapidly progressive (creseatic) glomeruli nephritis. Despite treatment with steroids and immunosuppressives, his kidney function continued to worsen and clinical dialysis needed to be instituted.

If this patient's ultrasonogram had demonstrated kidneys smaller than 7 cm, his course would have been considered chronic and less amenable to specific diagnosis or therapy. If the first urinalysis had not shown casts, repeated efforts to find them would be worth the extra time.

Conclusion

The incidence of many varieties of renal disease is increasing, and the primary care physician is the first to be consulted by many of the patients involved. The Rules of Three enhance facility of evaluation and often enable early intervention, noninvasive examination, and potential salvage of the remaining renal parenchyma. It is hoped that more noninvasive tools and improved treatments for renal disease will be developed. Advances such as these would enable more specific causative management and less renal injury, without attendant complications.

Suggested Reading

1. Chen MY, Zagoria RJ. Can noncontrast helical CT replace intravenous urography for evaluation of patients with acute urinary tract colic? *J Emerg Med.* 1999; 17:299-303.

2. Chevalier RL, Klahr S. Therapeutic approaches in obstructive uropathy. *Semin Nephrol.* 1998; 18: 652-655.

3. CPC: Acute renal failure in a 21-year-old woman. *Am J Med.* 1997;103:318-327.

4. Klahr S, Miller SB. Acute oliguria. *N Engl J Med.* 1998;338:671-675.

5. Michel DM, Kelly CJ. Acute interstitial nephritis. *J Am Soc Nephrol.* 1998;9:506-515.

6. Nolan CR, Anderson RJ. Hospital-acquired acute renal failure. *J Am Soc Nephrol.* 1998;9:710-718.

7. Thadhani R, Pascual M, Bonventre JV. Acute renal failure. *N Engl J Med.* 1996;334:1448-1460.

13. Drug-Induced Acute Renal Failure

Recognizing and Treating Prerenal, Postrenal, and Pseudorenal Injury

Drug-induced acute renal failure (ARF) has become a common cause of morbidity and mortality. It is essential that primary care physicians be familiar with the risk factors and presentation of this condition, since early recognition, appropriate prophylaxis, and dose adjustment or discontinuation of nephrotoxic drugs may prevent serious renal complications. Table 13-1 summarizes the main causes and precipitating factors of ARF.

Although the risk of drug-induced renal insufficiency in healthy persons is practically nonexistent, it ranks among the major causes of ARF in vulnerable patients. A number of commonly prescribed and over-the-counter medications — NSAIDs, for example — can cause abrupt renal insufficiency in a vulnerable person. Moreover, drugs are responsible for up to 20% of cases of ARF among inpatients and 15% of renal injuries among patients in intensive care units.

In one study of ARF among inpatients, 37% of the episodes had surgical causes, 27% had medical causes, 15% resulted from sepsis, and as many as 21% were caused by a variety of nephrotoxic substances.[2] Hospital-acquired ARF substantially increases both patient mortality and overall costs; in one study, the risk of death increased 6.2-fold, and the median duration of hospitalization rose from 13 to 23 days.

In this article, we will review three major types of drug-induced ARF, using case presentations to highlight diagnosis and management. We will approach drug-induced ARF in the same systematic fashion as ARF of any cause. To set the stage for these case studies, we will briefly review — and illustrate — the mechanisms underlying drug-induced renal insufficiency.

We will then consider specific drugs that mediate prerenal and postrenal injury. Finally, we will review drugs that may elevate creatinine levels without changing renal function. Intrarenal toxicity will be addressed in the following chapter.

Table 13-1. Causes of acute renal failure

Cause	Precipitating factor
Prerenal (reversible and irreversible)*	
Hypovolemic states	Hemorrhage, GI tract and third space losses
Reduced cardiac output	Cardiogenic shock
Systemic hypotension	Sepsis, hepatic failure, antihypertensives
Increased renovascular resistance	Hepatic failure, alpha-agonists
Decreased intrarenal arteriolar resistance	NSAIDs, angiotensin-converting enzyme inhibitors (given when decreased effective plasma volume or renal artery stenosis are present)
Arterial or venous obstruction Rhabdomyolysis Intravascular hemolysis	Thrombosis, emboli
Renal	
Acute tubular necrosis	Prerenal causes and nephrotoxins
Acute cortical necrosis	Profound shock, especially with abruptio placentae
Glomerular disease	Rapidly progressive and postinfectious glomerulonephritis
Acute interstitial nephritis	Drugs, infection, myeloma, lymphoma, granuloma, uric acid
Small-vessel disease	Vasculitis, toxemia of pregnancy, hemolytic-uremic syndrome, malignant hypertension
Postrenal	
Obstruction	Tumors, bleeding, fibrosis, stones

*All prerenal causes may eventuate in acute tubular necrosis.

Prerenal Drug-induced ARF

Although renal tissue constitutes a mere 0.4% of total body mass, the kidney receives 20% to 25% of the cardiac output. Renal blood flow is precisely regulated by responsive vascular smooth muscle in afferent and efferent glomerular vessels and by endothelial-active substances, such as prostaglandins, nitric oxide, and angiotensin II, as well as by the adrenergic nervous system. A disturbance in any of these regulators could lead to a change in renal perfusion, intraglomerular pressure, and ultimately glomerular filtration.

ACE Inhibitor-induced Prerenal Insufficiency

A very commonly prescribed class of medications, angiotensin-converting enzyme (ACE) inhibitors are an important pharmacologic cause of prerenal ARF. (The other class is NSAIDs, discussed below.) ACE inhibitors can reduce intraglomerular pressure; under normal physiologic conditions, this does not substantially decrease the glomerular filtration rate (GFR), but it may protect glomeruli from hydraulic or hyperfiltration injury. Such injuries result from exposure of the glomerular capillary bed to excessive, protracted elevations in pressure. This pharmacologic action enables ACE inhibitors to reduce proteinuria in patients with the nephrotic syndrome and to slow the progression of renal disease in diabetic patients with proteinuria. However, hypoperfusion of the renal vasculature mediated by either volume loss or ineffective circulation increases renin and angiotensin II levels. This increase in vasoconstrictors compensates for circulatory inadequacy by raising blood pressure, while GFR is maintained by efferent arteriolar constriction.

Since ACE inhibitors decrease angiotensin II levels, they produce efferent arteriolar dilatation in high-renin states. Under these circumstances, intraglomerular pressure would be reduced, which could lead to a decline in GFR. Patients who are most sensitive to the adverse renal effects of ACE inhibitors are those most dependent on the renin-angiotensin system: patients who are volume-contracted or those who have "ineffective" circulation.

Volume contraction and ineffective circulating volume are both sensed by the kidney — appropriately — as a threat to survival. The decreased renal perfusion in these states increases renin synthesis and release, which ultimately supports blood pressure and circulation through the generation of angiotensin II. The rise in angiotensin II levels results in constriction of the efferent arteriole, which maintains glomerular hydraulic pressure in the face of hypoperfusion. The inhibition of angiotensin I to II conversion may lower blood pressure and precipitously decrease the GFR.

Correcting volume or improving the ineffective circulation (eg, by reducing afterload appropriately, by ensuring adequate left ventricular filling pressures, and by treating ischemia if present), along with discontinuing the ACE inhibitor, will improve the GFR and the acute renal insufficiency. When the azotemia and congestive heart failure (CHF) are treated and have resolved, ACE inhibitor therapy may be reinstituted at a lower dose with gradual, careful titrations (eg, captopril, 6.25 mg twice daily or enalapril, 2.5 to 5 mg/d to start).

Two case studies will illustrate the clinical implications in more detail.

CASE 13-1. ACE Inhibitor-induced ARF in association with CHF

History. A 64-year-old obese woman with a 15-year history of non-insulin-dependent diabetes mellitus, hypertension, and insulin resistance was hospitalized for increasing dyspnea. Her course had been complicated by diabetic retinopathy (treated by laser), microalbuminuria, and peripheral neuropathy. Her blood pressure had been reasonably controlled (130 to 140/84 to 95 mm Hg) with a diuretic (hydrochlorothiazide, 25 mg/d) and a calcium channel blocker (sustained-release diltiazem, 180 mg/d).

Physical examination. On admission, the patient's blood pressure was 160/90 mm Hg, pulse was 106 beats per minute and regular, and respiratory rate was 26 breaths per minute and labored; she was afebrile. Pertinent findings included jugular venous distention at 30 degrees;

Table 13-2. Oliguria: 'The rules of three'

Categories of oliguria

Postrenal

Prerenal

Renal (parenchymal insufficiency)

Noninvasive diagnostic tools

History and physical examination

Ultrasonography

Urinalysis with urinary electrolytes

Clinical maxims

All oliguria is considered obstructive until proved otherwise

A carefully done urinalysis, using a fresh specimen, is critical in the workup of every oliguric patient

Only after postrenal and prerenal causes are eliminated can the third category (parenchymal insufficiency) be pursued

---

bibasilar rales; left and right ventricular hypertrophy by palpation and a holosystolic apical murmur that increased with isometric hand grip (consistent with mitral regurgitation); mild hepatomegaly with some tenderness; peripheral edema; and symmetric peripheral neuropathy.

Laboratory data. The patient's glucose level was 220 mg/dL with normal serum electrolytes. Her blood urea nitrogen (BUN) level was 36 mg/dL; creatinine concentration was 1.3 mg/dL; hemoglobin, white blood cell and platelet counts were normal. Urinalysis showed 2+ glucose and protein on dipstick with a negative sediment.

Initial workup and treatment. Admission diagnosis was congestive heart failure (CHF), and ECG findings were consistent with left ventricular (LV) hypertrophy and sinus tachycardia. Normal enzyme (CPK-MB) values, troponins, and an ECG ruled out acute myocardial infarction. Echocardiographic results were consistent with biventricular global dysfunction, suggesting cardiomyopathy from small-vessel diabetic disease and moderate mitral regurgitation. The patient's LV ejection fraction was decreased (34%).

Angiotensin-converting enzyme (ACE) inhibitor therapy was begun with captopril, 25 mg three times a day, and furosemide, 80 mg/d. The patient's symptoms and signs of CHF resolved within 24 to 36 hours. However, approximately 72 hours later, the BUN level was 60 mg/dL, creatinine concentration was 2.6 mg/dL, and the patient showed signs of oliguria (urinary output of <400 mL over the preceding 24 hours).

Discussion. Even though this patient's azotemia worsened with the concurrent initiation of ACE inhibitor therapy (making this agent the likely nephrotoxin), renal failure should ideally be approached with the "rules of three" to ensure that other possible causes are not overlooked (Table 13-2). In this case, postrenal causes were eliminated by ultrasonography, which demonstrated no obstruction. Prerenal causes contributed to renal failure, since the administration of furosemide decreased LV filling pressures. The combination of compromised LV function and overdiuresis may have further contributed to a state of renal hypoperfusion. This then led to further deterioration of renal failure secondary to the ACE inhibitor. Furosemide, and the ACE inhibitor were discontinued, and the patient was allowed free access to fluids. The patient's BUN and creatinine returned to baseline. Reinstitution of ACE therapy did not adversely affect renal function.

Case 13-2: ACE Inhibitor-Induced ARF in Association With Renal Artery Stenosis

History. A 72-year-old man with known vascular disease and a long smoking history presented with refractory hypertension. Two months before, his blood pressure had been 180/115 mm Hg, and despite titration of a three-drug regimen (furosemide, 40 mg/d; sustained-release diltiazem, 90 mg twice daily; and terazosin, 10 mg/d), his blood pressure remained at 162/102 mm Hg.

Physical examination and laboratory data. Pertinent findings included a grade II hypertensive retinopathy, left ventricular hypertrophy by palpation, an S_4 gallop, and decreased peripheral pulses with the absence of dorsalis pedis and posterior tibial pulses. The blood urea nitrogen (BUN) level was 18 mg/dL, and the creatinine concentration was 1.5 mg/dL.

Treatment and outcome. The patient was started on enalapril, 10 mg/d, and a diuretic (hydrochlorothiazide, 25 mg/d). Three days later, he returned with symptoms of oliguria, including rising levels of BUN (40 mg/dL) and creatinine (2.9 mg/dL).

In this patient, the peripheral vascular disease, resistant hypertension, and mild azotemia suggest underlying ischemic nephropathy, a condition also characterized by renal artery stenosis and often nephrosclerosis. If the renal artery stenosis is bilateral and severe, or occurs in a solitary functioning kidney, the administration of an angiotensin-converting enzyme (ACE) inhibitor may lead to acute renal failure because of efferent arteriolar dilatation.

After this patient was admitted to the hospital, the ACE inhibitor was discontinued, and he was carefully given IV fluids (0.9% sodium chloride at 125 mL/h). Over the next 72 hours, his creatinine level decreased to 2 mg/dL. A renal arteriogram obtained 2 days later showed bilateral renal artery stenosis (85% right, 90% left) that was subsequently corrected with bilateral renal artery angioplasty.

Discussion. The development of acute renal failure during ACE inhibitor therapy should lead to the discontinuation of the medication and a determination of whether volume contraction, ineffective circulation (as with congestive heart failure), or renal vascular disease is responsible for the renal failure.

NSAID-induced Prerenal Insufficiency

Although the precise incidence is difficult to determine, NSAIDs appear to be one of the most common causes of drug-induced prerenal ARF. Like ACE inhibitors, NSAIDs may also cause hemodynamically mediated renal failure within days to weeks of the onset of therapy. Ketorolac may induce renal injury earlier than other NSAIDs (5 or more days). Since NSAIDs inhibit the formation of vasodilating prostaglandins through their action on cyclooxygenase, they block the afferent arteriolar compensatory mechanism for decreased renal blood flow (dilation in response to decreased blood pressure or perfusion), resulting in afferent arteriolar constriction. Whereas ACE inhibitors may dilate the efferent arteriole and thus decrease intraglomerular pressure, NSAIDs cause constriction of the afferent arteriole with the same net effect — decreased intraglomerular pressure with a resulting fall in GFR (Figure 13-1).

A recent study of risk factors for NSAID-induced ARF demonstrated that most affected patients were men older than 50 years who had conditions associated with poor renal perfusion. These conditions included diuretic use with volume contraction, vomiting/diarrhea, serum albumin level less than 3.1 g/dL, GI bleeding, and CHF. Active sodium retention as a response to either volume contraction or ineffective circulating volume seems to render the renal vasculature extremely sensitive to the adverse effects of NSAIDs. Theoretically, agents with little or no effect on renal prostaglandin synthesis would be less likely to induce these types of changes in renal perfusion. Nonacetylated salicylates (salsalate, choline magnesium trisalicylate, diflunisal), sulindac, and nabumetone may have less effect on renal prostaglandin synthesis. However, controlled studies have not been done to confirm these benefits.

Another study demonstrated that the greatest risk factor for NSAID-induced ARF was a recent hospitalization for other illnesses. This suggests that sicker patients are more likely to require an intact prostaglandin-mediated renal dilatation during circulatory stresses. In this study, the relation between NSAID use and ARF was dose-dependent. As expected, ARF resolved when the NSAIDs were stopped. Conditions such as CHF, hypotension, ascites, nephrosis, and cirrhosis may make patients vulnerable to NSAID-induced renal failure and should prompt a cautious approach with NSAID use or, if necessary, complete avoidance. Table 13-3 highlights predisposing conditions and other features of NSAID-induced hemodynamic deterioration of renal function.

NSAID-induced and ACE inhibitor-induced prerenal failure have similar presentations and warrant equal caution. Patients with ineffective circulating volume or volume contraction are in a high renin-angiotensin II state. The kidney maintains its perfusion and filtration despite angiotensin II-induced vasoconstriction by compensating with vasodilatory prostaglandins. NSAIDs inhibit prostaglandin synthesis and thus may provoke a precipitous decline in both renal blood flow and GFR. This effect is reversible with discontinuation of the medication, as well as with correction of either volume contraction or ineffective circulating volume.

Table 13-2. NSAID-induced hemodynamic deterioration of renal function

Predisposing conditions
  Extracellular fluid volume depletion
  Congestive heart failure
  Cirrhosis (particularly with ascites)
  Nephrotic syndrome
  Underlying renal disease
  Third space fluid sequestration
  Diuretic therapy
  Advanced age

Additional features
  Usually is precipitated by higher doses
  Course may be oliguric or nonoliguric
  Usually reversible and usually does not require dialysis

CASE 13-3: NSAID-Induced ARF in Association With CHF and GI Bleeding

History. A 70-year-old woman who had chronic crippling rheumatoid arthritis was hospitalized with congestive heart failure (CHF). She had a history of an anterior wall myocardial infarction with ischemic cardiomyopathy and a left ventricular ejection fraction of 30%. She had been discharged about 3 weeks previously after treatment for CHF. She had gained approximately 10 lb since her last outpatient visit and had experienced increasing dyspnea with orthopnea over the prior 10 days. She had used NSAIDs regularly to combat arthritic pain.

Physical examination. The patient's blood pressure was 170/90 mm Hg; pulse was 110 beats per minute and regular, and respiratory rate was 26 breaths per minute and labored. Examination findings included jugular venous distention at 30 degrees, bibasilar rates, a holosystolic mitral regurgitation murmur, and an S_3 gallop. Peripheral edema was present. Treatment for the patient's CHF included nitrates, furosemide, and administration of captopril (6.25 mg twice daily).

Laboratory data. The patient's stool guaiac test was positive, and the hemoglobin level had decreased from 12.6 g/dL on her previous admission to 9.2 g/dL. She complained of joint pains, and NSAID therapy was restarted. On admission, her blood urea nitrogen and creatinine levels were 28 mg/dL and 1.7 mg/dL, respectively. She became progressively oliguric over the next 48 hours, and the creatinine level doubled.

Discussion. This patient clearly demonstrates the typical risk factors for NSAID-induced renal insufficiency: advanced age, recent hospitalization, CHF, and GI bleeding. She also manifested a dose-dependent response, since as an outpatient she had been taking NSAIDs without supervision. In addition, the simultaneous use of captopril may have had a synergistic adverse renal hemodynamic effect with the NSAIDs.

Stopping the NSAID agent improved the orthopnea. Her renal function gradually returned to normal. Cox-2 agents have similar effects on the kidney.

Postrenal Drug-induced ARF

Drugs may cause renal tubular obstruction either by direct precipitation or as a result of a process in which tissue breakdown products literally plug the renal tubules. The drug involved is usually one that is less soluble in an acidic urine. Therefore, alkalinization of urine and hydration are the cornerstones of management and prevention of a variety of failures of the postrenal type.

Drugs commonly associated with postrenal ARF in at-risk patients (ie, those with volume contraction or azotemia) include the older sulfonamides, acetazolamide, methotrexate, acyclovir, and massive IV doses of vitamin C (which is metabolized to oxalic acid). These drugs are highly insoluble in acidic urine; patients taking them should be advised to drink plenty of water. Alkalinization of urine is probably not necessary to prevent precipitation if adequate hydration is achieved, but if renal insufficiency occurs, sodium bicarbonate should be administered to increase the solubility of the substance. An increase in urinary pH from 5 to 6 has an exponential effect on urine solubility.

Other classes of drugs that may be associated with postrenal ARF include antineoplastic agents and 3-hydroxy-3-methylglutaryl coenzyme A (HMG-CoA) reductase inhibitors.

Antineoplastic agents. Uric acid nephropathy — a precipation nephropathy — may occur following antineoplastic therapy for cancer with a large tumor load (eg, lymphoma). This therapy may cause rapid cellular destruction and the release of intracellular components, including uric acid. The result is precipitation of uric acid crystals in the renal tubules and acute renal failure.

Preventive measures consist of pretreatment hydration, urinary alkalinization, and the administration of allopurinol. In fact, preventive measures have been so successful that this type of renal failure has become quite rare. The use of uricosuric agents, such as probenecid for the treatment of gout, may also precipitate uric acid nephropathy. The uricosuric effect of these drugs is most prominent at the onset of therapy, so it is prudent to give patients 3 to 7.5 g of sodium bicarbon-ate per day (or its equivalent) and recommend plenty of water intake until serum uric acid levels normalize and tophaceous deposits disappear.

HMG-CoA reductase inhibitors. This class of drugs is the one most commonly associated with drug-induced rhabdomyolysis, which can result in ARF secondary to intratubular precipitation of myoglobin. Since the concomitant use of erythromycin, cyclosporine, gemfibrozil, or niacin and an HMG-CoA reductase inhibitor increases the incidence of rhabdomyolysis, these drug combinations should be avoided. ARF induced by HMG-CoA reductase inhibitors is particularly prevalent in solid organ transplant patients. If rhabdomyolysis occurs, hydration and alkalinization of the urine should be implemented.

Pseudorenal Failure

Finally, remember that drugs may produce elevations in blood urea nitrogen (BUN) or creatinine that do not indicate a real change in renal function. Corticosteroids and tetracycline may increase protein catabo-lism so that BUN levels may increase while the serum creatinine concen-trations and GFR remain unchanged.

Since creatinine is not only filtered but also secreted, organic bases that compete for secretion of creatinine can cause an elevation in serum levels without a change in glomerular filtration. Cimetidine is an organic base known to interact with creatinine in this way. Because of their higher potency, the other H_2 blockers have minimal effects on creatinine secretion. Trimethoprim may also falsely elevate serum creatinine levels by inhibiting the tubular secretion of creatinine.

In patients with good renal function, inhibition of creatinine secretion rarely causes a significant increase in serum concentrations. However, as renal function declines, secretion of creatinine becomes a larger compo-nent of creatinine clearance. The result is a more profound effect on serum concentrations in patients with borderline renal dynfunction.

Cephalosporin antibiotics (eg, cefoxitin, cefazolin, and cefotetan) are known to interfere with the Jaffé test for measuring creatinine, although this interaction does not generally occur with the newer creatinine measurement methods. Flucytosine may cause false elevations in serum creatinine values when an iminohydrolase enzymatic assay is used to measure creatinine. Flucytosine does not interfere with the Jaffé reaction.

Suggested Reading

1. Aronoff GR. Therapeutic implications associated with renal studies of nabumetone. *J Rheumatol.* 1992;19(suppl 36):25-31.

2. Bilheimer DW. Long-term clinical tolerance of lovastatin and simvastatin. *Cardiology.* 1990;77(suppl 4):58-65.

3. Brenner BM. *Brenner & Rector's the Kidney.* ed. Philadelphia: WB Saunders Company; 1996:1699.

4. Chapman AB, Gabow PA, Schrier RW. Reversible renal failure associated with angiotensin-converting enzyme inhibitors in polycystic kidney disease. *Ann Intern Med.* 1991;115:769-773.

5. Cortin HL, Bonventre JV. Factors influencing survival in acute renal failure. *Semin Dial.* 1989;2:220.

6. Curry SC, Chang D, Connor D. Drug and toxin-induced rhabdomyolysis. *Ann Emerg Med.* 1989;18:1068-1084.

7. Feldman HJ, Kinman JL, Berlin JA, et al. Parenteral ketorolac: the risk for acute renal failure. *Ann Intern Med.* 1997;126:193-199.

8. Gallego FLA, Pascual J, Garcia-Martin FG, et al. Prognosis of acute tubular necrosis: an extended prospectively controlled study. *Nephron.* 1993;63:21-31.

9. Gutthan SP, Rodriguez LG, Raiford DS, et al. Non-steroidal anti-inflammatory drugs and the risk of hospitalization for acute renal failure. *Arch Intern Med.* 1996;156:2433-2439.

10. Lawton JM, Conway LT, Crosson JT, et al. Acute oxalate nephropathy after massive ascorbic acid administration. *Arch Intern Med.* 1985;45:950-951.

11. Lewis EJ, Hunsicker LG, Bain RP, Rhode RD. The effect of angiotensin-converting enzyme inhibition on diabetic nephropathy. *N Engl J Med.* 1993;329:1456-1462.

12. Rutecki GW, Whittier FC. The rules of three in oliguria: how to use this technique for evaluation. *Consultant.* 1993;33(1):43-59.

13. Shankel SW, Johnson DC, Clark PS, et al. Acute renal failure and glomerulopathy caused by non-steroidal anti-inflammatory drugs. *Arch Intern Med.* 1992;152:986-990.

14. Shustennan N, Strom BL, Murray TG, et al. Risk factors and outcome of hospital-acquired acute renal failure. *Am J Med.* 1987;83:65-71.

15. Stillman MT, Schlesinger PA. Nonsteroidal anti-inflammatory drug nephrotoxicity. *Arch Intern Med.* 1990;150:268-270.

16. Whitworth JA, Lawrence JR, eds. *Textbook of Renal Disease.* 2nd ed. London: Churchill Livingstone Inc;1994:303.

14. Drug-Induced Acute Renal Failure
Keys to Recognizing and Treating Intrarenal Toxicity

Although drug-induced acute renal failure (ARF) has been a common cause of morbidity and mortality, early recognition, appropriate prophylaxis, and dose adjustment or discontinuation may prevent catastrophic complications. It is therefore critical that primary care physicians be familiar with the risk factors and presentations of this condition.

Here we will review the largest category of drug-related ARF — intrarenal toxicity — and some of its primary causes, including acute tubular necrosis and acute interstitial nephritis. We will also present two case studies that illustrate the clinical features of these forms of drug-induced ARF.

Acute Tubular Necrosis

Nephrotoxic injury to the tubular cells can result from ischemia or pharmacologic activity. Early signs of nephrotoxicity include subclinical tubular proteinuria and enzymuria and disturbances in the renal processing of electrolytes. Tubular injury manifests as an elevation in the fractional excretion of sodium, which may increase from less than 1% to more than 3%. Nephrotoxicity and other conditions that reduce renal perfusion (for example, bleeding with volume contraction and ineffective circulatory states) can decrease the glomerular filtration rate by decreasing intraglomerular pressure. If the offending agent is not removed, the kidney may eventually become ischemic, and a prerenal state will deteriorate to frank renal failure.

ARF may be induced by a number of agents commonly used by primary care physicians, including aminoglycoside antibiotics, amphotericin B, and radiocontrast media (Table 14-2). We will review these agents and outline a strategy for preventing nephrotoxicity.

Aminoglycosides. Nephrotoxic injury is the primary adverse effect associated with aminoglycoside antibiotics. The incidence of this effect increased from about 2% in 1969, when these agents were introduced, to about 20% in 1993. The percentage of patients who experience nephrotoxicity rises with duration of therapy, reaching almost 50% after

14 or more days. Although the exact mechanism of aminoglycoside nephrotoxicity is unknown, the drug may accumulate and bind with lysosomal phospholipids within tubular cells, thus creating cell damage.

Assessing the risk. Although a number of studies have attempted to assess risk factors associated with aminoglycoside-induced acute tubular necrosis, there are two flaws common to these studies that make interpretation difficult. The first is defining nephrotoxicity simply as a decrease in creatinine clearance, even though this decrease may not be clinically significant. For example, in some studies toxicity was defined as an increase in the serum creatinine value of 40% or more, which means that a patient with a baseline creatinine level of 0.6 mg/dL that increases to 0.9 mg/dL was considered to have significant renal injury.

Another flaw involves the methods used to relate serum concentrations of an aminoglycoside to nephrotoxicity. Early studies classified patients with minimally elevated trough concentrations of an aminoglycoside as suffering from nephrotoxity. However, since aminoglycosides are eliminated by the kidney, patients in whom renal insufficiency develops during therapy have increased trough concentrations of animoglycosides simply as a result of decreased renal elimination. Subsequent studies that monitored serum concentrations serially from the outset of therapy were not able to establish a clear correlation between trough concentrations and renal injury. An excellent review by McCormack and Jewesson addresses this issue.

Reducing the risk. Several strategies may be employed to reduce the risk of aminoglycoside toxicity. These include avoiding aminoglycoside use in patients with known risk factors (Table 14-2), prescribing the shortest therapeutic course possible, monitoring serum concentrations, and using once-daily dosing.

Although specific serum concentrations have not been clearly correlated with renal injury, preventing accumulation of the drug may nevertheless minimize toxicity. When nephrotoxicity occurs, the aminoglycoside concentration increases before the serum creatinine level does; it thus serves as a marker for renal deterioration.

Several studies have demonstrated a statistically significant decrease in nephrotoxicity with once-daily administration of aminoglycosides, compared with the traditional BID or TID regimen. Aminoglycocides kill microorganisms in a concentration-dependent fashion. So, for example, once-daily administration of 4 to 5 mg/kg of gentamicin or tobramycin makes possible peak concentrations two or three times higher than traditional dosing and allows trough concentrations to fall to zero every 24 hours.

Table 14-1. Selected agents commonly associated with acute tubular necrosis

Anti-infectious drugs
- Acyclovir
- Aminoglycosides
- Amphotericin B
- Foscarnet
- Pentamidine

Anti-inflammatory and immunosuppressive medications
- Chemotherapeutic agents
- Cisplatin
- Cyclosporine
- Ifosfamide
- NSAIDs

Radiocontrast media

With the introduction of the newer broad-spectrum antibiotics, aminoglycosides are rarely indicated as the sole therapy for serious infections. They are usually added to a Beta-lactam regimen; the combination acts synergistically on both gram-positive and gram-negative organisms. The use of aminoglycosides for the entire 10 to 14 day course of antibiotic therapy is therefore usually not necessary. Instead, to help minimize the possibility of renal failure, combination therapy can be used for 3 to 5 days or until the patient shows signs of clinical improvement. The patient may then be switched to a regimen with less nephrotoxicity after antibiotic sensitivities return.

Radiocontrast Media

Radiocontrast media-associated ARF is more likely to occur when renal damage is already present, especially if there is concomitant diabetes mellitus. Table 14-3 lists the most common risk factors. The precise incidence is difficult to determine, but it is between 1% and 30%, depending on the number of risk factors present. Among patients with radiocon-trast media-associated ARF, there is nearly a fivefold increase in mortality, compared with patients who are given radiocontrast media but in whom ARF does not develop.

Radiocontrast media are classified as either high-osmolar or low-osmolar agents. High-osmolar agents are ionic and have an osmolality of 1,500 to 2,400 mOsm, or about 5 to 10 times that of plasma. The newer low-osmolar agents are nonionic and have an osmolality that is only 2 or 3 times that of plasma. Theoretically, the use of low-osmolar agents should reduce the incidence of nephrotoxicity seen with the high-osmolar agents. Initial trials were only able to demonstrate a reduced incidence of minor adverse reactions. One meta-analysis and one prospective study indicate that contrast nephrotoxicity may be mitigated in patients with preexisting renal insufficiency when low-osmolar agents are used.

In addition, low-osmolar agents cost approximately 10 times more than high-osmolar agents. Since there is no evidence of a reduction in nephrotoxic reactions with these agents in patients with normal renal function, their use should be reserved for patients at especially high risk not only for renal failure but also for any potentially serious complications.

Current recommendations suggest that hydration with 0.45% saline (1 mL/kg of body weight) for 12 hours before the procedure will provide protection against contrast-mediated renal injury in those at risk (Table 14-4).

Table 14-2. Risk factors for renal toxicity from aminoglycosides
Preexisting renal insufficiency
Dehydration/Volume depletion
Advanced age
Liver disease
Potassium depletion
Endotoxemia
Shock
Other nephrotoxins
Sustained elevated serum aminoglycoside concentrations
Past multiple courses of aminoglycosides
Frequent dosing
Prolonged duration of therapy

Case 14-1. A Diabetic Patient with Impaired Renal Function

History and laboratory date. A 41-year-old man with a 16-year history of insulin-dependent diabetes mellitus presented to the hospital with angina. Diabetic complications included mild, nonproliferative diabetic retinopathy and albuminuria (2.5 g in 24-hour urine specimen) that was being treated with ACEI. His blood urea nitrogen (BUN) level was 18 mg/dL, and his creatinine level was 1.4 mg/dL. (One year previously, his BUN and creatinine levels were 14 mg/dL and 1 mg/dL, respectively.) An ECG did not show acute changes but did have voltage criteria for left ventricular hypertrophy. Enzyme levels (of CPK-MB and troponin-A) did not suggest acute ischemic cardiac injury. Exercise thallium test results were consistent with ischemia. Cardiac catheterization was planned, and the cardiologist asked for advice concerning the potential for contrast injury in this diabetic patient with underlying renal disease.

Table 14-3. Risk factors for renal toxicity from radiocontrast media
Preexisting renal insufficiency
Diabetes mellitus (especially with renal insufficiency)
Dehydration/Volume depletion
Congestive heart failure
Advanced age
High dose of radiocontrast medium
Myeloma (if accompanied by volume contraction, hypercalcemia, or renal insufficiency)

Discussion. Patients who have impaired renal function resulting from diabetic renal disease are at greatest risk for contrast-mediated renal injury. Volume repletion before the administration of radiocontrast agents is the most important prophylactic measure in this group. An IV infusion of 5% dextrose and 0.45% sodium chloride at a rate of 1 mL/kg/h should be started in preparation for the procedure (12 hours beforehand, if possible). Since this patient is at high risk for contrast-mediated renal injury, a nonionic contrast medium, at the lowest dose possible, is recommended.

Because of the glucose load, the patient should have his serum glucose monitored and insulin adjusted as necessary. Urinary output should be monitored after the procedure (hourly initially), with continued volume replacement for at least 24 hours. Since no further contrast administration will be required after catheterization, the risk of renal injury is likely to disappear after the first day.

Since nephrotoxic agents may increase the likelihood of renal injury, ACEI should be discontinued temporarily and other such medications (eg, NSAIDs, aminoglycosides) should be avoided. Metformin is contraindicated in patients with renal insufficiency and should be discontinued before contrast studies in patients with non-insulin-dependent diabetes mellitus. The administration of dopamine, furosemide, or mannitol in low doses may also increase the risk of renal injury in patients with diabetes by inducing volume depletion.

Amphotericin B

The era of AIDS and other immunosuppressive conditions has seen a dramatic increase in systemic fungal infections and the parenteral use of amphotericin B. The incidence of amphotericin B-associated renal injury depends on the cumulative dose; it reaches 80% with a total dose of more than 4 g. Amphotericin B is thought to stimulate tubuloglomerular feedback, which in turn causes afferent arteriolar constriction and decreased renal blood flow, rendering the kidney ischemic and eventually inducing ARF. The recently available liposomal formulations of amphotericin B may accumulate preferentially in organs of the reticuloendothelial system rather than in the kidneys, and thus be protective against renal injury.

Sodium depletion is the most important risk factor for nephrotoxic injury; this has led to the common practice of saline loading both before and during drug administration, as long as there is no contraindication (Table 14-4). Consider also the sodium content of concurrent drugs patients may be taking. For example, a typical regimen of ticarcillin will deliver approximately 78 mEq of sodium per day, which is the equivalent of approximately 500 mL of normal saline. Similar precautions and prophylaxis should be considered with other nephrotoxic anti-infectious agents, such a acyclovir, pentamidine, and foscarnet.

Acute Interstitial Nephritis

This condition accounts for up to 15% of all cases of ARF. Most varieties of acute tubulo-interstitial injury are mediated by immunologic mechanisms. The pathology of acute interstitial nephritis involves a humoral or cell-mediated hypersensitivity response to pharmacologic agents. Drugs and their metabolites can serve as haptens that bind to proteins, which leads to the formation of immunogenic complexes. Drug-specific antibodies produced by B lymphocytes and other inflammatory cells then infiltrate the renal interstitium, causing peritubular inflammation and tubular injury within minutes to hours of exposure to the drug. T lymphocytes may also be involved in a cell-mediated immune reaction that can develop over a longer period (days to weeks) after the initial drug exposure.

Assessment and management. Acute interstitial nephritis can occur at any time during the initial or subsequent course of therapy with an offending drug. Patients who experience this response to medication have so-called immune response genes associated with a particular susceptibility to this type of acute renal injury. Prompt recognition of acute interstitial nephritis and discontinuation of the offending agent are crucial, since neglect of these steps may lead to chronic renal failure and dialysis.

Although many drugs have been implicated in the development of acute interstitial nephritis, relatively few have been frequently associated with the condition (Table 14-5). These include antibiotics such as methicillin, generic penicillin and ampicillin, the sulfonamides, and rifampin.

Signs of acute interstitial nephritis, such as fever, eosinophilia, rash, hematuria, proteinuria, sterile pyuria, oliguria, and eosinophiluria, appear approximately 10 to 20 days after initiation of therapy. These signs may be absent, although hematuria, proteinuria, sterile pyuria, and eosinophilia are observed often. About three quarters of patients are febrile, but a rash is seen in only 25%.

Many patients recover with removal of the offending agent; the likelihood of complete recovery appears to be inversely proportional to

---

Table 14-4. Sodium loading procedure to prevent nephrotoxicity from amphotericin B

- 1 L of 0.9% sodium chloride infused over 1 hour before each dose
  OR
- 500 mL of 0.9% sodium chloride given before and after each dose

the duration of renal failure. The use of corticosteroids in patients who do not improve rapidly is controversial. Small trials have been unable to demonstrate that their use alters outcome, although they may shorten the time to recovery of renal function. A typical regimen would be prednisone, 40 to 60 mg/d.

Acute interstitial nephritis that occurs secondary to NSAID use has a very different clinical picture than that induced by other drugs. The interstitial lesion typically appears after several months to a year of use; this delayed time to development of renal dysfunction is characteristic of a cell-mediated immune response. Systemic manifestations of a hypersensitivity response are present in only one of five patients who have this complication. Most patients respond to the removal of the offending NSAID.

Case 14-2. A Woman With Arthritis and Oliguria and Recent-Onset Hypertension

History. A 70-year-old woman with a history of degenerative arthritis presented to her physician with oliguria and recent-onset hypertension. She had had an uncomplicated right hip replacement 18 months previously, and her arthritis pain medication had been changed to fenoprofen from another NSAID approximately 6 weeks ago. She had noted a decrease in urine volume, orthopnea, and lower-extremity edema.

Physical examination. The patient's blood pressure was 180/100 mm Hg; her pulse was 110 beats per minute and regular; her respiratory rate was 22 per minute; and she had a temperature of 37.2^0 C $(99^0$ F). The patient was in mild respiratory distress but not otherwise uncomfortable. There was no evidence of rash. Pertinent findings included sinus tachycardia with an S_3 gallop, bibasilar rales, and a 2+ peripheral edema.

Laboratory data. The patient's serum electrolyte levels were sodium,

Table 14-5. Drugs associated with acute interstitial nephritis

Antibiotics
    Penicillins
    Rifampin
    Sulfonamides
    Vancomycin
    Ciprofloxacin
    Cephalosporins
    Erythromycin
    Minocycline
    Trimethoprim-sulfamethoxazole
    Ethambutol
NSAIDs
Diuretics
    Thiazides
    Furosemide
    Triamterene
Miscellaneous
    Captopril
    Cimetidine
    Ranitidine
    Phenobarbital
    Phenindione
    Phenytoin
    Allopurinol
    Interferon
    Interleukin-2
    Anti-CD4 antibody
    Acyclovir

136 mEq/L; potassium, 5 mEq/L; chloride, 100 mEq/L; and bicarbonate, 20 mEq/L. Her blood urea nitrogen (BUN) level was 52 mg/dL, and her creatinine level was 4.7 mg/dL. The renal insufficiency and oliguria were approached with the **Rules of Three** (Table 12-1). An ultrasonogram demonstrated that the kidneys measured 9.8 and 9.4 cm and that there was no obstruction. A chest film showed mild congestive heart failure.

These results suggested that neither a postrenal state nor volume depletion was responsible for the oliguria. A urinalysis showed 4+ protein on dipstick, and sediment contained hyaline and finely granular and coarsely granular casts. A 24-hour urine specimen showed > 3 g of protein in 600 mL.

Discussion. The concurrence of fenoprofen use, renal insufficiency, and glomerular proteinuria made the combination of intrarenal injury from minimal change disease and acute interstitial nephritis the most likely cause of acute renal failure. A percutaneous renal biopsy confirmed the diagnosis. The fenoprofen was discontinued, and the patient's renal function stabilized over approximately 5 days, with peak BUN and creatinine levels of 80 mg/dL and 7.6 mg/dL, respectively. One dialysis treatment was required because of fluid overload. The patient's BUN and creatinine levels then decreased to a baseline level of 18 mg/dL and 1.5 mg/dL, respectively.

Glomerulopathies

This group of glomerular diseases is generally immune complex-mediated and not associated with drug toxicity; however, four drug-induced lesions have been identified: membranous glomerulonephritis, minimal change disease, focal segmental glomerulosclerosis, and membranoproliferative glomerulonephritis. With the possible exception of focal segmental glomerulosclerosis from heroin use, the drug-related glomerulopathies are reversible once the drug is discontinued. Therefore, a careful medication history is essential, especially in patients with proteinuria. Be sure to ask specifically about NSAID use.

The rare patient in whom drug-induced glomerular disease develops presents with proteinuria, edema, and nephrotic syndrome. Quantitative urinary protein may be greater than 3 g in 24-hour specimens.

Membranous glomerulonephritis (membranous nephropathy). This is the most common drug-induced glomerular lesion; it results from the deposition of immune complexes along glomerular capillary loops. Parenteral gold, which may be used to treat rheumatoid arthritis, is the agent usually implicated; the incidence of gold-induced membranous glomerulonephritis is between 1% and 10%. Penicillamine, captopril, and NSAIDs may also be implicated.

A recent study retrospectively identified 125 patients with the early stages of the disorder. Of those patients, 29 were taking NSAIDs at the time the nephrotic syndrome developed and 13 met the criteria for NSAID-induced membranous nephropathy.

Minimal change disease. This condition can be caused by drugs such as NSAIDs, ampicillin, rifampin, phenytoin, and lithium. The glomerulopathy of NSAIDs may be accompanied by acute interstitial nephritis and usually resolves when the offending NSAID is discontinued.

Focal segmental glomerulosclerosis. This condition can occur in long-term heroin users as a reaction either to the heroin itself or to other injected contaminants (eg, talc). It is usually irreversible.

Membranoproliferative glomerulonephritis. This condition is associated rarely with nifedipine, penicillamine, and chlorpropamide. In a few patients, hydralazine may induce a syndrome simulating systemic lupus erythematosus.

Suggested Reading

1. Barrett BJ. Contrast nephrotoxicity. *J Am Soc Nephrol.* 1994;5:1237-1251.

2. Barrett BJ, Carlisle EJ. Meta-analysis of the relative nephrotoxicity of high and low osmolality iodinated contrast media. *Radiology* 1993; 188: 171-178.

3. Brenner BM, ed. *Brenner & Rector's the Kidney.* 5th ed. Philadelphia: WB Saunders Company;1996.

4. Freeman CD, Strayer AH. Mega-analysis of meta-analysis: an examination of meta-analysis with an emphasis on once-daily aminoglycoside comparative trial. *Pharmacotherapy.* 1996;16:1093-1102.

5. Gallis HA, Drew RH, Pickard WW. Amphotericin B: 30 years of clinical experience. *Rev Infect Dis.* 1990;12:308-329.

6. Hall CL. Gold nephropathy. *Nephron.* 1988;50:265-272.

7. Hatala R, Dinh T, Cook DJ. Once daily aminoglycoside dosing in immunocompetent adults: a meta-analysis. *Ann Intern Med.* 1996; 124:717-725.

8. Hiemenz JW, Walsh JT. Lipid formulations of amphotericin B: recent progress and future directions. *Clin Infect Dis.* 1996;22(suppl):S133-S144.

9. Lawrence V, Matthai W, Hartmaier S. Comparative safety of high-osmolality and low-osmolality radiographic contrast agents. *Invest Radiol.* 1992;27:2-28.

10. McCormack JP, Jewesson PJ. A critical reevaluation of the 'therapeutic range' of aminoglycosides. *Clin Infect Dis.* 1992;14:320-339.

11. Murray KM, Keane WR. Review of drug-induced acute interstitial nephritis. *Pharmacotherapy.*1992;12:462-467.

12. Radford MG, Holley KE, Grande JP, et al. Reversible membranous nephropathy associated with the use of nonsteroidal anti-inflammatory drugs. *JAMA.* 1996;276:466-469.

13. Rapp RP, Gubbins PO, Evans ME. Amphotericin B lipid complex. *Ann Pharmacother.* 1997; 31:1174-1186.

14. Rudnick MR, Goldfarb S, Wexler L, et al. Nephrotoxicity of ionic and nonionic contrast media in 1196 patients: a randomized trial. *Kidney Int.* 1995;47:254-261.

15. Rutecki GW, Whittier FC. The rules of three in oliguria: how to use this technique for evaluation. *Consultant.* 1993;33(1):43-59.

16. Solomon R, Werner C. Mann D, et al. Effects of saline, mannitol, and furosemide on acute decreases in renal function induced by radiocontrast agents. *N Engl J Med.* 1994;331:1416-1420.

17. Steinberg EP, Moore RD, Powe NR, et al. Safety and cost effectiveness of high-osmolality as compared with low-osmolality contrast material in patients undergoing cardiac angiography. *N Engl J Med.* 1992;326:425-430.

18. Toto Rd. Review: acute tubulointerstitial nephritis. *Am J Med Sci.* 1990;299:392-410.

19. Zarama M, Abraham PA. Drug-induced renal disease. In: DiPiro JT, Talbert RL, Yee GC, et al, eds. *Pharmacotherapy: A Pathophysiologic Approach.* 3rd ed. Stamford, Conn: Appleton and Lange; 1997: 1007-1031.

INDEX